CURING EVERYDAY AILMENTS

The Natural Way

CURING
EVERYDAY
AILMENTS

The Natural Way

THE READER'S DIGEST ASSOCIATION LIMITED
LONDON NEW YORK SYDNEY MONTREAL

Curing Everyday Ailments the Natural Way

For Reader's Digest, London

Editor:
Caroline Boucher

Art Editor:
Kate Harris

Proofreader:
Barry Gage

For Reader's Digest General Books, London

Editorial Director:
Cortina Butler

Art Director:
Nick Clark

Executive Editor:
Julian Browne

Development Editor:
Ruth Binney

Publishing Projects Manager:
Alastair Holmes

Picture Resource Manager:
Martin Smith

Style Editor:
Ron Pankhurst

Book Production Manager:
Fiona McIntosh

Pre-press Manager:
Howard Reynolds

Senior Production Controller:
Sarah Fox

Pre-press Account Manager:
Penny Grose

Created by Gaia Books Ltd

Project Manager:
Cathy Meeus

Art Editor:
Malcolm Smythe

Copy Editors:
Lynn Bresler, Sarah Chapman

Proofreader:
Deirdre Clark

Designers:
Phil Gamble, Ann Thomson

Illustrators:
Hayward Art Group, Karen Hiscock, Aziz Khan, Ruth Lindsay, Sheilagh Noble, James G. Robins, Harry Titcombe

Photographic Direction:
Tania Volhard, Sara Mathews, Matt Moate

Photographers:
Ray Moller, Paul Forrester

Picture Researcher:
Jan Croot

Indexer:
Jill Ford

Production:
Lyn Kirby, Kate Gaudern

Managing Editor:
Pip Morgan

Direction:
Joss Pearson, Patrick Nugent

Project Management and Typesetting
Aardvark Editorial, Suffolk

Chief Medical Editor:
Dr. Penny Stanway MB BS

Consultants:
Stefan Ball (Flower Essences), Ann Gillanders (Reflexology), Robin Hayfield (Homeopathy), Paul Lundberg (Acupressure and Shiatsu), Robin Monro (Yoga), Roger Newman Turner (Naturopathy), Jane Rieck (Massage), Robert Stephen (Aromatherapy), Christine Steward (Herbalism)

Writers:
Jane Alexander, Chris McLaughlin, Ricki Ostrov, Anna Selby, Wendy Teasdill, Philip Wilkinson

About This Book

How can you relieve pain without drugs? What foods can you eat to reduce your cholesterol level? What can you take to help you sleep if you suffer from insomnia? To these and a whole host of other questions, *Curing Everyday Ailments the Natural Way* provides you with authoritative, easy-to-apply answers you can trust.

The basics of natural health

In the introductory chapter, "Maintaining Health the Natural Way", you will find important information about the kind of diet, lifestyle, and home environment you need to become healthy and to stay healthy. As well as providing general advice on using natural therapies safely, this chapter also tells you how to create your own natural medicine cabinet. This way, you will have on hand the main remedies you need to treat common minor ailments at home.

About the therapies

Part One: The Therapies familiarizes you with the various types of treatments recommended in this book. It describes the theories behind 10 major therapies that you can use at home, along with instructions in basic techniques and important general cautions. A range of additional therapies that cannot properly be undertaken without the help of a qualified therapist is described more concisely in the "Glossary of Therapies".

Treating ailments naturally

The heart of the book is *Part Two: Symptoms and Ailments*, arranged for easy reference in A to Z order. If you don't find a specific problem in the table of contents, check the general index, which will guide you to the appropriate article. In Part Two, you will discover the nature and possible causes of your disorder, how you can prevent it, and which natural treatments can be used for it. With this information, you can make up your own mind about which therapies to choose, according to your preferences and symptoms. Always check the general instructions and cautions on using a particular therapy in Part One before embarking on a treatment.

Getting medical help

At the end of each article you will find advice about when to consult a doctor instead of treating a disorder at home with natural therapies. In some cases, certain symptoms are noted as requiring medical help right away—for example, by calling 999 or going to an accident and emergency unit. Otherwise, make an appointment with your doctor at the earliest opportunity. It is impossible to address every possible combination of symptoms so readers should also use their own judgment and always seek their doctor's guidance for unexplained or worrisome symptoms.

Extending your understanding

Cross-references appear in the text where appropriate to guide you to further explanations elsewhere in the book. A box at the end of each article notes related topics. Unfamiliar terms used in the text can be looked up in the "Glossary of Terms". Organizations that you may want to contact for more detailed information about natural therapies are listed, along with their addresses, telephone numbers, and web sites, where available, in the "Resource Guide".

Conversion Chart
Spoons and Cups

Metric	Imperial
1.25ml	¼ teaspoon
2.5ml	½ teaspoon
5ml	1 teaspoon
10ml	2 teaspoons
15ml	1 tablespoon
30ml	2 tablespoons
45ml	3 tablespoons
60ml	¼ cup
125ml	½ cup
150ml	⅔ cup
175ml	¾ cup
250ml	1 cup

Caution: Remember that it is never wise to mix metric and imperial measurements in the same remedy as amounts given are not exact equivalents.

Contents

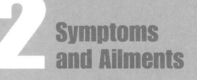

Maintaining Health the Natural Way

The various forms of natural medicine provide a gentle kind of health care that is becoming increasingly popular, though most people expect to combine it with orthodox medicine. Natural medicine offers long-term well-being because it acknowledges a person's lifestyle and treats the whole person—body, mind, and spirit—not just the symptoms of ill health.

Natural medicine is attracting increasing numbers of people. A recent survey showed that one person in five consulted a complementary or alternative therapist in the previous year, mostly for chronic problems, such as arthritis, back pain, and sleeping difficulties. Many more treat themselves with complementary or alternative remedies. This suggests that while orthodox medicine is claiming more success in tackling major health problems, such as cancer and heart disease, natural medicine is better able to satisfy other needs.

Why choose the natural way?

Healing based on natural remedies, home treatments, and lifestyle measures is considerably gentler and more user-friendly than taking potent medications. It also enables you to take responsibility for your everyday well-being while being free to consult a doctor or other health-care professional when appropriate. Perhaps most important, it acknowledges the good sense of maintaining the health of the entire person, rather than focusing on symptoms of disease, and it attempts to prevent, rather than simply treat, sickness.

Natural approaches to health recognize the body's own healing power and try to maximize or enhance it. They are also less likely than orthodox treatments to cause troublesome

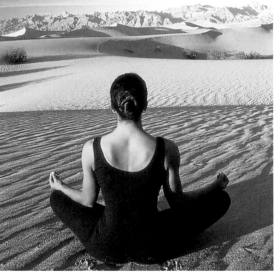

Harnessing your own healing power
Natural therapies, from acupressure to yoga, aim to utilize the body's inherent power of self-healing.

side effects. Each herbal remedy, for example, contains small amounts of several active ingredients, each of which tends to balance the actions of the others. This is in contrast to most prescription drugs, which typically contain a powerful dose of a single substance and therefore have the potential to unbalance the body chemistry and create new problems that may in turn necessitate further treatment.

Natural medicine places great emphasis on the important links between the body and mind. Scientific research provides an ever-increasing volume of evidence to substantiate this approach. A wealth of studies shows that patients who think positively and address any emotional problems tend to have improved outcomes in diseases ranging from arthritis to cancer. Brain and body are intimately linked by hormones, neurotransmitters (substances that help transmit messages between nerve cells), and other chemicals. Mood changes can affect the functioning of your immune system, your cardiovascular health, and the quality of your sleep. On the other hand, physical problems affect your happiness, alertness, and anxiety level. This explains why physical illness can often lead to mental distress and vice versa, and why physical therapies can alleviate mental illness and mind therapies may indeed encourage physical healing. A good example is laughter therapy (see p. 63). Seeing the funny side of life and laughing a lot can promote chemical changes in the body that may help to keep you well.

Choices for health

It is tempting, perhaps, to see conventional and natural medicine as irreconcilable opposites. But the reality is that many mainstream doctors are happy for patients to include natural approaches in their treatment. Similarly, reputable practitioners of complementary and alternative therapies recognize the importance of obtaining orthodox medical advice for all but minor ailments. Trying natural therapies does not have to imply excluding yourself from the undisputed benefits of "high-tech" medicine; instead it's a way of extending your treatment options. This "integrated" approach to health is discussed further on page 17.

The keys to healthy living

A good diet, regular exercise, and using strategies for managing stress are the main ways to maintain health naturally. Other important aids include fostering your relationships, making your home a healthy place in which to live, and avoiding damaging practices, such as smoking. Looking after yourself in this way encourages mental well-being and helps you protect every part of your body, from arteries to nerves, intestines to hormone-producing glands. It can also bolster your immune system, helping protect you from infections, allergies, and even cancer.

This introduction contains information about all these essential aspects of health maintenance, plus guidelines on selecting the natural therapies that will work best for you.

Eat well, be well

The food you eat is the source of the energy you need to fuel the activity of every cell in your body. It also provides the nutrients required for physical growth and repair and enables the body to produce the variety of substances, such as hormones, enzymes, and neurotransmitters, that are essential for normal body functioning.

Ideas about food have changed in recent years. Not so long ago, a widespread belief was that avoiding certain foods, such as fats, ensured a healthy diet. While reducing the excessive consumption of fats is still seen as important, greater emphasis is now placed on following a diet that contains a good balance of nutrient-rich foods. The "Healthy eating pyramid" on page 10 shows the proportions of different types of foods that most people need to achieve this balance.

Buying and preparing food

When you buy food, think about which items are best for your health. For example, favour poultry and fish over red meat, because red meat contains more saturated fat. Also favour cold-pressed oils that contain beneficial monounsaturated and polyunsaturated fats, rather than butter or other solid fats, which contain saturated fats. Select low-fat dairy products whenever you can. If available, choose organic foods, which are grown without pesticides, antibiotics, or growth-promoting hormones. Such foods are cultivated in ways that promote healthy growth and development, as well as disease resistance. Maximize nourishment by eating a high proportion of foods that have been processed as little as possible, such as whole grains and fresh fruit and vegetables.

Preserve the nutritional value of fresh foods by preparing them just before mealtimes. With organic foods, you should generally discard as little fruit and vegetable peel as possible. But if you eat non-organic produce, remember that any traces of insecticides, fungicides, or herbicides are most likely to be found in the peel or outer leaves. Clean produce carefully. Cook fruit and vegetables lightly to retain vitamins and minerals. If you fry, do so quickly, using fresh oil each time.

➤ *continued, p. 11*

Maintaining Health the Natural Way

Healthy eating pyramid
This illustrates the relative amount of each food group you should include in your daily diet. Make the foods at the base of the pyramid your staples and include only small quantities of the foods shown at the apex.

Sweets: Add sweetness to food, if necessary, with a little honey, maple syrup, or sugar. But try to make these ingredients only an occasional treat. Sweet foods provide quick energy and, sometimes, trace amounts of minerals.

Fats: Restrict your fat intake to no more than 30 percent of total calories. This includes fats "hidden" in other foods and those used for cooking. Favour vegetable fats (in nuts, seeds, whole grains, vegetables, cold-pressed vegetable oils) and fats from oily fish over fats in meat, eggs, and dairy products. Fats provide fatty acids that are vital for cell structure and contain fat-soluble vitamins.

Protein-rich foods: Eat four to six daily helpings. These foods include poultry, fish, eggs, low-fat dairy products, lean meat, nuts, beans, and bean products, such as tofu. Proteins are needed for cell growth and repair and for the production of antibodies, hormones, and enzymes.

Vegetables and fruit: Eat at least three to five daily helpings of vegetables and two to four of fruit. Include a variety of roots, tubers, stems, leaves, fruits, and seeds and pods. Choose fruit and vegetables of a range of colours (because different plant pigments offer different health benefits). These foods supply fibre, vitamins, minerals, and some essential fatty acids.

Complex carbohydrates: Eat 6 to 11 servings of unrefined starchy foods, such as rice, beans, root vegetables, bananas, and whole grains, or foods made from them (such as wholegrain bread, breakfast cereal, and pasta). Complex carbohydrates are a ready source of energy and contain vitamins and minerals.

Portion size

Protein
2–3 ounces of meat, fish, and poultry
1 egg
1 cup of milk or yogurt
1 1/2 ounces of hard cheese
1/2 cup of nuts or cooked beans or lentils

Vegetables and fruit
1/2 cup of non-leafy vegetables
1 cup of leafy vegetables
1 medium apple, orange, or pear
1/2 grapefruit or melon
1/2 cup of canned or stewed fruit

Carbohydrates
1 slice of bread
1 ounce of uncooked cereal
1/2 cup of cooked root vegetable, pasta, cereal, or rice

Supplementing your diet

Supplements are no substitute for eating well, and most of the time a healthy diet provides all the nutrients you need. Your body builds reserves of some nutrients. Body fat, for example, stores fat-soluble vitamins (vitamins A, D, E, and K). Calcium and many other minerals can move from your bones to wherever else they are needed in your body. This means that you need a certain amount of these nutrients over a period of some weeks or months, but a daily variation in intake does no harm. Some other nutrients, such as water-soluble vitamins (vitamins B and C), are not stored, so you need to replenish them every day. Several conditions make supplements advisable. For example, supplements can:

■ Provide vital nutrients during pregnancy and in later life.
■ Help prevent ill health from a lack of nutrients in the diet.
■ Help treat illnesses, such as infections, that increase the rate at which the body uses certain nutrients.
■ Help treat illnesses, such as arthritis, that respond to increased levels of particular nutrients.
■ Help prevent or treat cardiovascular disease and diabetes.

Reference Nutrient Intake (RNI)

Many supplement labels give the percentage of the RNI for certain nutrients in the product. The RNI is the amount of a nutrient that is enough to meet the needs of at least 97.5 percent of the population (though the amount recommended is higher than most people need). RNIs have largely replaced Recommended Daily Allowances (RDAs), defined as the quantities of nutrients most people need on a regular basis if they are to stay healthy. These figures do not allow for variations in requirements resulting from illness, and may vary for smokers or people taking medication. RNIs are meant to provide general guidelines rather than hard-and-fast rules. A therapist may therefore advise you to eat more than the RNI of some nutrients in order to help your body function at its best.

Product packaging suggests doses and indicates the percentage of the RNI ("Reference Nutrient Intake") or the RDA ("Recommended Daily Allowance") dietary allowance (see box below) per capsule or tablet. The best choice is often a general-purpose multiple vitamin and mineral supplement, or one devised for a particular problem or time of life, though sometimes supplements of individual nutrients are advisable. Some formulations are more efficiently utilized than others. Look for the following:

■ Calcium—with magnesium, zinc, and vitamin D.
■ Iron—with vitamin C and copper.
■ Magnesium—with calcium, phosphorus, and vitamin B_6.
■ Selenium—yeast-based selenium with vitamins A, C, and E.
■ Zinc—zinc gluconate (if for colds and flu) with vitamin A and copper.
■ Vitamin A—as mixed carotenoids (such as beta-carotene).
■ Vitamin B—as vitamin B complex.
■ Vitamin C—in a preparation with flavonoids (sometimes called bioflavonoids).
■ Vitamin E—with mixed tocopherols.

The average healthy person converts linoleic and alpha-linolenic acids, known as essential fatty acids (see "Key nutrients and foods", p. 12), into such important body chemicals as hormones, and prostaglandins, which regulate a number of body processes. Some people cannot convert essential fatty acids properly, and nutritionists may recommend for them supplements of evening primrose oil, linseed oil, or fish oil.

Another group of supplements that is gaining popularity comprises those containing one or more essential amino acids (the molecules that make up proteins). There are many different types of amino acids, and these play an important role in building and repairing body tissues. They are normally obtained from protein-rich foods in your diet. But as with other nutrients, a number of conditions may impair the body's

➤ *continued, p. 13*

Key nutrients and foods

Nutrient and its role	Common food sources	Nutrient and its role	Common food sources
Beta-carotene *Antioxidant made into vitamin A*	Yellow and orange vegetables and fruit, green leafy vegetables	**Magnesium** *Energy production, nerve function, insulin regulation*	Fish, shellfish, meat, wholegrain cereals, nuts, green leafy vegetables, mushrooms, seaweed, seeds, cocoa
Calcium *Bone and tooth maintenance, muscle and nerve function*	Milk and cheese, fish plus their edible bones, wholegrain cereals, legumes, nuts, green cabbage	**Phosphorus** *Bone and tooth maintenance*	Egg yolks, fish, shellfish, meat, wholegrain cereals, legumes, soy, milk products
Chromium *Blood-sugar regulation*	Cheese, wholegrain cereals	**Potassium** *Fluid balance, muscle function*	Wholegrain cereals, nuts, seeds, vegetables, fruit, cocoa
Copper *Iron absorption, energy utilization, nerve function*	Fish, legumes, green leafy vegetables, mushrooms, avocados, garlic, seaweed, nuts, cocoa	**Selenium** *Antioxidant*	Milk products, fish, meat, wholegrain cereals, legumes, green leafy vegetables, mushrooms, garlic
Essential fatty acids *Blood-fat regulation, hormone production*	Wholegrain cereals, legumes, nuts, seeds, cold-pressed vegetable oils, dark-green leafy vegetables	**Zinc** *Growth and reproduction, enzyme action, immune function*	Milk products, fish, shellfish, meat, wholegrain cereals, legumes, root vegetables, garlic, sprouted seeds
Fibre *Bowel function*	Wholegrain cereals, vegetables and legumes, fruit, nuts, seeds	**Vitamin A** *Skin, hair, and eye maintenance, immune function*	Milk products, eggs, fish, legumes, cold-pressed vegetable oils
Flavonoids *Antioxidant*	Wholegrain cereals, brightly coloured vegetables and fruit	**Vitamin B complex** *Healthy metabolism, nerve function*	Milk products, fish, meat, legumes, wholegrain cereals, green leafy vegetables, seeds, nuts
Folic acid *Red blood cell formation, healthy cell division*	Liver, wholegrain cereals, green leafy vegetables, fruit, nuts, yeast	**Vitamin C** *Blood-vessel strength, wound healing, antioxidant*	Citrus and most other fruit, broccoli, peppers, and most other vegetables
Iodine *Thyroid hormone formation*	Fish, shellfish, meat, wholegrain cereals, green leafy vegetables, peppers, seaweed, iodized salt	**Vitamin D** *Bone and tooth maintenance*	Milk products, egg yolks, seaweed, nuts, oily fish, fish-liver oils
Iron *Oxygen transport*	Eggs, shellfish, meat, wholegrain cereals, legumes, green leafy vegetables, seaweed, dates, figs, raisins, seeds, cocoa	**Vitamin E** *Antioxidant, muscle function, red blood cell formation*	Vegetable oils, eggs, fish, wholegrain cereals, lentils, beans, nuts, seeds

ability to absorb or utilize them. People whose diet may contain a limited range of proteins, such as vegans, should consider taking a supplement that supplies a wide range of amino acids. Supplements of individual amino acids should not be taken for more than a few weeks without medical supervision. Amino acids should not be given to children without medical advice.

Get active, get fit

Exercise helps keep your bones, joints, and muscles in good condition. It can also boost your metabolism, counter stress, and help fight depression. To maintain good health, get the three types of exercise described on pages 13–14. Exercise regularly. Aim for a half hour of aerobic exercise, whether you do it all at once or in five- to ten-minute sessions throughout the day, for five days a week. If you no longer exercise, try to determine why you have become inactive and choose a new programme of exercise that more closely meets your needs and preferences. Consider all your personal circumstances: your ability, whether you like competition, whether you prefer to be alone or in a group, at home or away, indoors or outside. If motivation is a problem, consider consulting a professional trainer, who can tailor exercises to your needs and help you achieve your goals.

Exercising safely

- Choose an activity of suitable intensity for you.
- Stay within the target heart rate guidelines for your age (see box, p. 14).
- Warm up and cool down for 10 minutes before and after exercise.
- Consult your doctor if you are new to exercise, have an existing medical condition or back problem, are pregnant, or if you don't feel well after exercise.
- Get expert advice from a doctor or physical therapist after any exercise-induced injury.

Aerobic exercise

This type of exercise works large groups of muscles. If it is sufficiently intense, it raises your heart rate enough to build cardiovascular fitness. Examples include walking fast enough to make you warm, running, swimming, and playing tennis. Aerobic exercise also raises the blood levels of natural, hormone-like chemicals such as endorphins, inducing a feeling of well-being; it speeds up circulation, helping keep the arteries, veins, and heart healthy; and it raises the body's metabolic rate (the rate at which cells burn energy), which helps prevent you from putting on weight. In summary, aerobic exercise improves lung capacity and circulation, promotes heart health, boosts immunity, benefits digestion, helps maintain joint health, fosters weight control, and lifts the spirits.

Exercise that raises the heart rate to between 50 and 75 percent of your maximum rate (approximately 220 minus your age) is classified as moderate intensity, and that which raises the heart rate to a higher level is considered high intensity. For most people, regular moderate-intensity exercise provides all the health benefits they need. High-intensity exercise is mainly for serious athletes and those who wish to achieve above-average levels of fitness. It should not be attempted by those who are new to exercise.

Check your pulse periodically during exercise sessions. Unless you're more advanced, don't let your pulse rise above the moderate-intensity limit for your age (see box, p. 14). If you have trouble taking your pulse, use this rule of thumb for gentler forms of exercise, such as walking: If you can talk while exercising, you're not overdoing it; if you can sing, you may need to exert more effort.

Strength training

This type of exercise involves working individual muscles or muscle groups. Strength training can be done with or without weights or other loads. Examples include carrying an infant, lifting weights in a gym, and any repeated muscle

Your target heart rate

When starting exercise, aim to keep your pulse at the lower end of the moderate-intensity range, indicated below. Build up to a higher level gradually. (These figures are based on average maximum heart rates; they may vary.)

Age	Lower rate	Upper rate
	(beats per minute)	
20	100	150
30	95	142
40	90	135
50	85	127
60	80	120
70	75	112

work, such as rowing or cycling (which also provides aerobic exercise). Strengthening your muscles can prevent lower back pain, ease osteoarthritis, increase bone density, encourage weight loss, foster agility and balance, and lessen the risk of muscle injury. Do some of this sort of exercise at least twice a week.

Stretching

This type of exercise lengthens muscles to their full natural extent, promoting flexibility. Whether you stretch before aerobic exercise or strength training, or perform yoga or another activity that limbers the muscles and joints, you'll help prepare your muscles for activity, prevent

Fat-burning exercise
Regular aerobic exercise helps you get rid of excess fat and keeps you fit and healthy.

and relieve muscle stiffness after exercise, reduce the risk of muscle injury occurring, and prevent or ease back pain and repetitive strain injury.

Health hazards

A good diet, regular exercise, and stress management are at the core of any disease prevention programme. Nevertheless, many other areas of life under your control have an impact on health. For instance, it is important to not smoke—or at least cut down—and to consume only moderate amounts of alcohol. Also, make sure you protect yourself against the sun's ultraviolet rays when necessary, while also getting sufficient exposure to natural light. In addition, eliminate or reduce toxins, allergens, and contaminants in your home.

Cigarettes and alcohol

Smoking and/or drinking can adversely affect health and the more you indulge in either habit, the greater the risks.

Smoking: The addictive nature of nicotine encourages ongoing exposure to the harmful tars and gases in tobacco smoke. Breathing the smoke from other people's cigarettes or cigars—passive smoking—also carries risks, although of a lower order. Health problems linked to smoking include the following:

- The destruction of 25 milligrams of vitamin C per cigarette.
- Poor wound healing and premature skin aging.
- Asthma, bronchitis, and emphysema.

Common threats
Smoking and excessive drinking are standard practice in some social situations. However, they carry many health risks.

- Mouth, lung, and other cancers.
- Rheumatoid arthritis.
- Anxiety and depression.
- Deafness.
- Ulcerative colitis.
- Arterial disease.
- Osteoporosis.

In addition, smoking or passive smoking by a pregnant woman can lead to her baby having a low birth weight. Parental smoking before and after the birth increases the risk of sudden infant death syndrome (SIDS, or cot death).

Alcohol: Drinking in moderation and at appropriate times has little or no negative effect and may even be beneficial to your heart, perhaps because it raises the levels of HDL—good—cholesterol. However:

- Driving or undertaking other potentially hazardous operations after drinking alcohol increases the risk of accidents.
- Overindulgence can cause a hangover.
- Drinking too much in any one session intensifies your current mood and in the long run has a depressant effect.
- Alcohol consumption disrupts normal sleep patterns.
- Addiction can lead to social problems (including violence), malnutrition, high blood pressure, gastritis, liver damage and reduced liver function, and mouth and other cancers.
- Drinking alcohol during pregnancy can affect the health of the unborn baby.

Once consumed, alcohol is absorbed into the bloodstream. The liver gradually breaks down the circulating alcohol into other substances and eventually clears alcohol from the blood completely—unless you have drunk more alcohol in the meantime. The more alcohol you drink, the longer it takes for the liver to clear it from your bloodstream. Drinking one unit of alcohol (a glass of wine, a glass of average-strength beer, or a single measure of spirits) raises the blood-alcohol level by 15 milligrams per 100 millilitres. It takes an hour for the average person's body to clear a drink containing one unit of alcohol. Women are more susceptible than men to the damaging effects of alcohol because they absorb it faster and develop higher levels in their blood.

Giving up or cutting down: If you want to smoke or drink less, or stop completely:

- Acknowledge the pros and cons of both your habit and being a non-smoker or non-drinker.
- Look at alternative, non-damaging ways of enjoying yourself and managing stress.
- Forgive yourself for any lapses, then resume abstinence.
- Accept any need for support, then find that help.
For further advice, see "Addictions", pp. 76–77.

Light exposure

Growing scientific evidence indicates that good health depends partially on adequate exposure to the various wavelengths of electromagnetic radiation in natural light. Daily exposure to bright light affects the pineal gland and hypothalamus and alters the levels of various hormones and neurotransmitters. Too little exposure can lead to seasonal affective disorder (SAD) and the symptoms of jet lag.

The proportions of the different wavelengths in light form its "spectral balance". The spectral balance of sunlight changes with the time, season, weather, and distance from the equator, as well as the level of air pollution and any passage through glass (in windows or spectacles), both of which reduce the proportion of ultraviolet light. Different types of electric light have different spectral balances, and these can affect physical and mental health. Full-spectrum bulbs are available that mimic the afternoon sun; these may be worth investing in for some of your light fixtures, especially if you suffer from SAD. Exposing your skin to a certain amount (15 or 20 minutes) of direct sunlight boosts your production of vitamin D and "feel-good" chemicals such as endorphins.

Be very careful, however, not to overdo it. Too much of the sun's ultraviolet light can cause skin cancer, including malignant melanoma, and increases the likelihood of cataracts. To protect yourself, follow the advice on page 350, and also wear sunglasses in strong sun.

Making your home a healthy place

Some home comforts can be hazardous to your health. Fitted carpets, for example, harbour dust mites, which can trigger asthma and eczema in some people. Dust mites also flourish in the warm, still air encouraged by central heating and well-insulated homes. Electrical gadgets create electromagnetic fields, which at close range are suspected of increasing the risk of cancer. Make your home safer by adopting as many as possible of the following strategies:

- Introduce enough fresh air (especially if someone smokes).
- Avoid extremes of temperature and humidity.
- Keep some houseplants to freshen the air. Plants can absorb certain potentially toxic chemicals. Among the most efficient plants are spider plants, chrysanthemums, coconut palms, weeping figs, gerberas, and dracaenas.
- Do not use household cleaners and other chemicals in spray form; these encourage asthma in susceptible people.
- Whenever possible, substitute such substances as bicarbonate of soda and vinegar for harsh household cleansers.
- Have adequate lighting.
- Keep sound levels within reasonable limits.
- Do not sit close to the sides or back of a television or computer for long periods.
- Follow instructions with care when using potentially poisonous household chemicals (including solvents, glues, drain cleaners, and pesticides).
- Get expert advice when removing old lead paint.
- Take care of such hazards as loose stair carpeting and trailing electrical cords.
- Do not turn up your boiler thermostat too high.

- Minimize formaldehyde exposure by avoiding MDF (medium-density fibreboard) furniture (coating all exposed surfaces with varnish or polyurethane) and by painting MDF-panelled walls with paint designed to absorb formaldehyde emissions.
- Install smoke detectors and consider a carbon-monoxide detector, especially if you have a gas stove or a garage attached to your home.
- Have your home checked for radon gas.

Using natural therapies

Many people already treat ailments with natural remedies and therapies, and a lot more are interested in finding out what to use and how. Turning to natural therapies is not a substitute for a doctor. Most people who use alternative therapies, such as homeopathy, rely on their regular doctor for diagnosis and for health care in cases of serious illness. But increasing numbers of mainstream doctors are recognizing that certain complementary therapies have much to offer in treating specific ailments (for example, osteopathy or chiropractic for back pain), and they are likely to refer their patients to the appropriate complementary practitioner.

Home use

The natural approach often works well for common, everyday ailments, from coughs and colds to upset stomachs. There are so many therapies available that the choice can seem baffling. Use Part One of this book to find out about specific therapies, and consult the ailment entries in Part Two to learn which therapies are best for your problem.

Some therapies are especially well suited to specific types of ailments. Posture and movement training, for example, often improves such problems as back pain and tension headaches, while breathing exercises may shorten panic attacks and prevent asthma. But many therapies can be used to treat a wide variety of conditions.

You should also be guided by your personal preferences when selecting a natural therapy. Some people prefer therapies based on exercise; others favour those based on medicines. A therapy is more likely to work for you if you are comfortable with it. Remember that caring for yourself in a kind and thoughtful way is often the most important form of therapy.

Health professionals: an integrated approach

Consider yourself and your doctor or other health-care provider as a team. Play your part by maintaining a healthy lifestyle and treating yourself with natural remedies and therapies when appropriate. In the past, many doctors based most of their treatments on drugs and ignored traditional

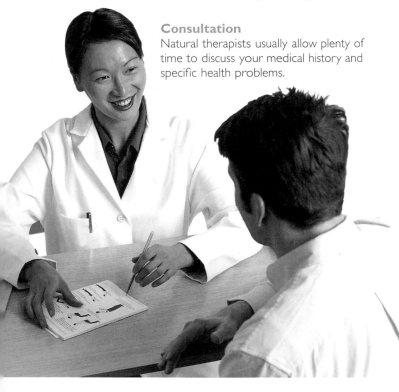

Consultation
Natural therapists usually allow plenty of time to discuss your medical history and specific health problems.

Choosing a natural therapist

Look in the ailment section in Part Two of this book to find out which therapies are recommended for your complaint, then read about the therapies in Part One to see if you find them appealing.

Finding a therapist
Once you have decided on a therapy, select a therapist by:
- Asking your doctor, friends, or neighbours for their recommendations.
- Scanning the register of therapists compiled by that therapy's national or local professional association.
- Checking with hospital-based referral lines.

Interviewing a therapist
Your first visit should be an exploratory one in which you:
- Ask the therapist about his or her treatments and personal approach.
- Ask about the therapist's training and qualifications.
- See if you feel comfortable with the person.
- Enquire about the therapist's experience, professional support, and insurance.
- To be doubly safe, check his or her credentials with the relevant professional association.

Working with your therapist
- Aim to work as a team with your therapist for the good of your health by sharing all relevant information and following a sensible programme of treatment.
- Be aware that your therapist may one day want to discuss your ailment with your doctor. However, he or she will seek your permission first.

When to beware
- Do not continue with a course of treatment if you feel uneasy or doubt the person's skill.
- Be suspicious of any therapist who promises a complete cure, emphasizes unusual or expensive testing, or promotes the sale of large amounts of costly supplements or equipment.

therapies. However, attitudes are now changing, with more and more doctors regaining an interest in older, natural healing methods. Preventive lifestyle measures, such as regular exercise, stress management, and a good diet, are well accepted, as are some complementary therapies.

Nowadays doctors work in conjunction with other health providers, including nurses and health visitors. These health professionals are not medical doctors, but they are licensed to provide primary care and to carry out certain procedures and tests, such as monitoring long-term conditions. They are becoming increasingly popular as a useful source of sound advice on problems which are not life-threatening, and they will know when to advise you to consult a doctor for a further evaluation of your condition.

Doctors and other health providers may also work with complementary or alternative therapists, such as naturopaths, aromatherapists, and osteopaths. Some medical centres offer a blend of orthodox and complementary medicine, which is known as integrated health care. This allows doctors and complementary practitioners to work alongside each other and so provide access to a greater variety of healing skills and to in-depth knowledge and experience of more specialized areas, such as nutrition and stress counselling. As communication and cooperation increase in this way, the exchange of ideas can enrich both the practitioners and the patients.

You should inform your doctor if you are undergoing other therapy at the same time as medical treatment, in case the two types of treatment interact and cause complications. See your doctor for:
■ Screening tests, routine checkups, immunizations, guidance on diet and lifestyle, and contraception.
■ Ante-natal care.
■ Advice on ailments. See the individual entries in Part Two of this book for more specific information and guidance on when to ask for help.

The natural remedy cabinet

On the following pages you will find lists of natural health products—food supplements, medicines, and basic equipment—that you may want to keep at home. Some of these items you may already have to hand; others you will have to buy. Resist the temptation to purchase large numbers of natural medicines. Most of these products have a limited shelf life, so keep only those supplements and remedies you will use every day and those that you think will be helpful for common ailments or first aid. Buy or make anything else only when you need it, so you won't have to discard expired products. Make sure that remedies remain clearly labelled and that implements are cleaned after each use. Purchase replacements before they are needed.

The uses described for the remedies in this section are for general reference only. Refer to the appropriate section in Part One of this book for cautions concerning each type of natural therapy. Check the appropriate entry in Part Two for more detailed guidance on using natural remedies for specific ailments.

Safe storage
Natural remedies should be kept in the same way as other kinds of medicines: in a cool place (or the refrigerator, when indicated) and away from children, sunlight, and humidity.

Vitamin, mineral, and other supplements

Keep your basic stock to a minimum. The following products are useful for many families:

- **Multiple vitamin and mineral supplement:** Particularly helpful if your eating habits are poor. Special vitamin and mineral supplements are available for certain times of life (as for pregnancy).
- **Borage (starflower) or evening primrose oil:** A good source of omega-6 fatty acids if your diet or digestion is poor. Also recommended if you suffer from premenstrual syndrome.
- **Fish-oil capsules:** A source of omega-3 fatty acids.
- **Vitamin C:** 500-milligram vitamin C tablets with flavonoids (as vitamin C complex or as separate items) may help at the first sign of a viral or bacterial infection, for inflammatory conditions, for daily use if you are a smoker, or if your diet is lacking in vitamin C.
- **Vitamin E:** Helps protect against heart disease; enhances the immune system; aids skin healing. Especially good for people with circulatory disorders.

Flower essences

If you are frequently affected by mental or physical distress and you find that flower remedies help, stock those that most closely match your emotions. The following are good standbys for most people:

- **Olive:** For stress.
- **Rescue Remedy:** For emotional shock or physical trauma, such as may follow a fall or other injury.

Herbal remedies

Select those remedies that you consider appropriate for your family's needs. For safety concerns, see pp. 34–37.

- **Aloe vera gel:** For burns or to soothe irritated skin (use a leaf from a houseplant or a commercial preparation).
- **Arnica cream:** For bruises, sprains, and chilblains (distinct from the homeopathic cream of the same name).
- **Black cohosh or dong quai:** For menstrual and menopausal problems.
- **Chamomile leaves or teabags:** For anxiety; anxiety-provoked wind, nausea, indigestion, diarrhoea, and sleep problems; itching; menstrual pain; and infections.
- **Comfrey ointment:** For sprains and strains when the skin is not broken.
- **Cramp bark tincture or dried bark:** For menstrual pain and leg cramps.
- **Echinacea tincture:** For boosting resistance to infection and to counter allergic reactions and inflammation.
- **Elderberry extract:** For colds and influenza.
- **Elderflowers:** For fevers and allergic rhinitis.
- **Fennel seeds:** For wind and indigestion.
- **Ginger (dried):** For nausea, wind, and cold extremities.
- **Myrrh tincture:** For mouth ulcers, gum disease, and a sore throat.
- **Slippery elm:** For indigestion and splinters.
- **Willow bark:** For inflammation.
- **Witch hazel (distilled):** For cuts, scrapes, bruises, insect bites, varicose veins, and haemorrhoids.

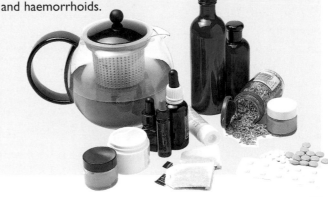

Aromatherapy oils

Select from the following list the essential oils that you think will be most useful. You will also need cold-pressed vegetable, nut, or seed oil for diluting essential oils other than lavender, tea tree, and clove (see p. 29).

- **Clove:** For toothache.
- **Eucalyptus:** For respiratory infections and fungal skin infections.
- **Lavender:** For burns, insect bites, cold sores, aching muscles, weakness, anxiety, headaches, depression, sleep problems, and splinters.
- **Peppermint:** For upper respiratory infections, fever, irritable bowel syndrome, and cuts and scrapes.
- **Roman chamomile:** For fever, insomnia, and inflammatory conditions.
- **Tea tree oil:** For bacterial and fungal skin infections, and vaginal yeast infections.

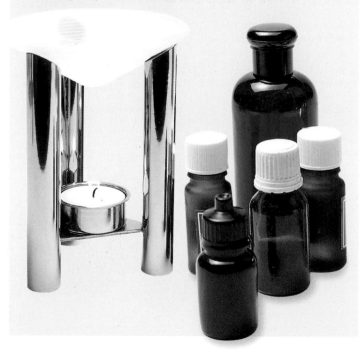

Homeopathic remedies

These remedies need to be selected according to the precise nature of your symptoms. However, the following are applicable to a wide range of conditions and are good to have on hand. Choose 6c potency (see "Less is more", p. 39) for remedies taken by mouth.

- **Aconite:** For sudden onset of high fever.
- **Belladonna:** For headache.
- **Coffea:** For insomnia.
- **Hypercal (St. John's wort and calendula):** As cream or topical solution for chilblains and other skin problems.
- **Ipecacuanha:** For nausea.
- **Ledum:** For puncture wounds.
- **Nux vomica:** For nausea.
- **Rhus toxicodendron:** For sprains and strains.

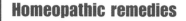

Useful items

- **Glass droppers:** For measuring essential oils.
- **Skin brush or loofah:** For boosting circulation if you have cold hands and feet or varicose veins.
- **Hot-water bottle or heatable pad:** For relieving muscle aches and abdominal cramps.
- **Thermometer:** For measuring temperature (the ear type is the most accurate and easy to use).
- **Ice pack:** For bruises and sprains.

Kitchen-cabinet basics

Many foods, herbs, and other products normally kept in the kitchen can also be used to treat common ailments. The following examples are helpful for a variety of illnesses. Check appropriate articles in Part Two for advice on correct usage.

- **Apple-cider vinegar:** For arthritis, colds, fungal skin infections, hair and scalp problems, indigestion, insect bites and stings, itching.
- **Bicarbonate of soda:** For allergic skin reactions, cuts and scrapes, gum disease, insect bites.
- **Carrots:** For appetite loss, coughs, weak nails, threadworms. As a broth, for dermatitis and dry or chapped skin (apply cooled carrot broth to the skin).
- **Bag of frozen peas:** To use as an ice pack.
- **Extra-virgin olive oil:** For diluting essential oils and for treating ear wax, earache, dermatitis, indigestion, sore lips.
- **Garlic (raw):** For cold hands and feet, earache, fungal skin infections, bacterial and viral infections, urinary-tract infections, threadworms, warts.

- **Ginger (fresh):** For colds, fever, indigestion, nausea, menstrual cramps, poor circulation (cold hands and feet).
- **Honey:** For colds, coughs, fever, allergic rhinitis, splinters (in a poultice), skin infections, and for sweetening herbal teas.
- **Lemons:** For corns, fever, indigestion, infections, sore throat.
- **Mustard seeds or powder:** For cold hands and feet and to make warming footbaths to treat colds.
- **Onions:** For upper respiratory-tract infections, wind, insect bites and stings, warts.
- **Prunes or figs:** For constipation.
- **Salt:** For diarrhoea (to make a sugar-salt mixture, see p. 290), earache, gum disease, mouth ulcers, sore throat.

First-aid kit

Gather the following items for first aid and keep them all in one place, such as a suitably marked box or cupboard so that you know where to find what you need in an emergency.

- **Sterile cotton wool:** For cleaning wounds.
- **Clean cotton fabric:** For making compresses.
- **Stretch bandages (such as crêpe ones) and safety pins:** For supporting sprained muscles.
- **Gauze bandages:** For holding dressings in place.
- **Surgical adhesive tape:** For securing gauze bandages or holding dressings in place.
- **Large triangular piece of cotton fabric:** For making a sling.
- **Non-adherent sterile dressings:** For cuts and burns.
- **Adhesive plasters:** For minor cuts and scrapes.
- **Scissors**
- **Eye bath:** For bathing irritated or infected eyes.

- **Sterile eye-pad with ties:** For eye injuries.
- **Tweezers:** For removing splinters, bees' sting sacs, and ticks.

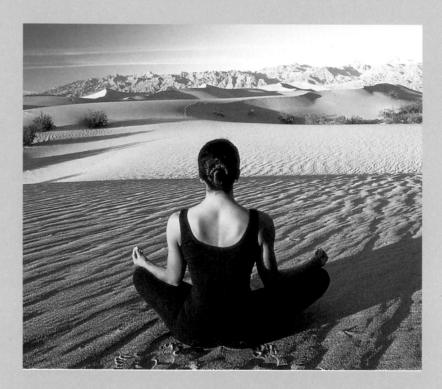

1 The Therapies

In this part of the book you will find information on the general principles behind a wide range of popular natural therapies. These remedies may serve as a gentle adjunct to the treatment and advice provided by your doctor and other health-care professionals. However, before using any of the therapies at home or consulting a natural therapist, be sure to familiarize yourself with the basic techniques and, above all, take note of any special precautions.

Acupressure and Shiatsu

These two therapies are based on the theory that a form of energy flows through the body along channels called meridians. Pressing key points on the meridians is believed to regulate the flow of energy, thereby improving health. Acupressure is the technique for applying pressure to these points. Shiatsu uses acupressure together with a range of other methods to affect the energy flow.

Acupressure has its roots in ancient Chinese medicine, which views the health of the body in terms of the level and flow of energy along the meridians, said to run up and down the body from head to toe. In Chinese medicine, this vital energy is called qi (pronounced "chee" and sometimes written "chi"). Imbalances or blockages in the flow of qi around the body are said to lead to ill health, so Chinese physicians may treat disease by regulating the flow of qi. One way in which they do this is by pressing on certain points on the body where the meridians are said to come close to the skin. Pressing on these points is believed to strengthen or disperse qi, according to the condition being treated and the type of pressure used.

Palm pressure
With shiatsu, before working specific points, you may move along the limbs, pressing with your whole hand.

Practitioners in China have been working with pressure points for thousands of years, using acupuncture (see p. 58) as well as acupressure to affect the flow of qi. During the sixth century, Buddhist monks took this form of therapy to Japan, where it also became popular. Much more recently, in the 1920s, Japanese doctors developed shiatsu, a therapy that combines finger pressure on the pressure points (known by shiatsu practitioners as *tsubos*) with such techniques as palm pressure and muscle stretches.

Consulting a professional

A professional shiatsu or acupressure practitioner will first assess your state of health. Besides examining you and asking you questions about your medical history, lifestyle, and diet, he or she will study your muscle and skin tone and listen to your voice and breathing.

For treatment, you usually lie on a mat on the floor. The therapist will apply pressure to certain key points on your body and may also perform massage or muscle stretches at the same time.

As the therapist works, he or she uses the sense of touch to

➢ continued, p. 26

Meridians and pressure points

The meridians are invisible pathways along which energy is said to flow around the body. Pressing points along them is thought to regulate energy. There are corresponding meridians and therefore acupressure points on both sides of the body (right). The illustrations, right, show points on one side of the body. Two meridians, called the Governing and Conception Vessels, lie along the body's midline.

Although practitioners work with several hundred points, the figures here show only the main points used in this book. Their technical names are included so that you can relate them to the instructions given for specific ailments. While some points have Chinese names, most consist simply of a letter or letters, which refer to the organ or system that the point is thought to affect, and a number indicating its position on the meridian. In Chinese medicine the functions of the organs are viewed very differently from the way they are in Western medicine. For example, the point LI (Large Intestine) 4 is used not only to regulate the intestine, but also to treat headaches, colds, and sinus trouble. The Heart Protector, linked to the pericardium, has a wide influence on all the chest organs. The Triple Heater is an "organ" that has a function—distributing energy—but no physical form.

Yin and yang

In Chinese medicine all energy is divided into two complementary aspects: yin and yang. In simplified terms, yang is active and "masculine" and yin is passive and "feminine". Each meridian is classified as either yin or yang. The Governing Vessel meridian controls the yang meridians and the Conception Vessel controls the yin meridians.

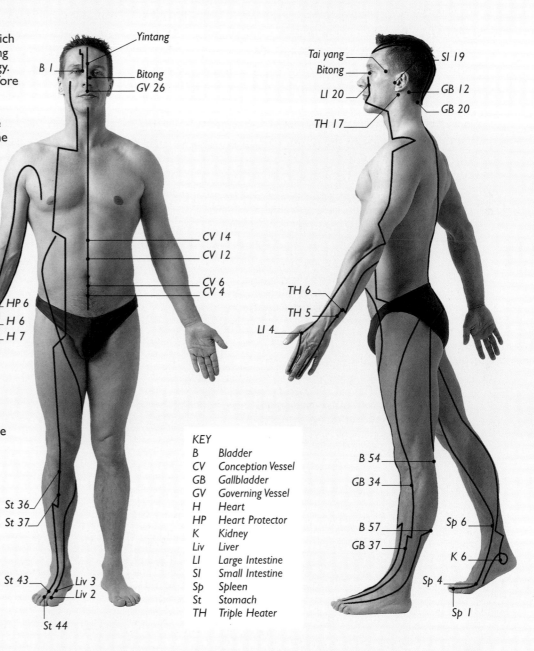

Yintang
B 1
Bitong
GV 26
CV 14
CV 12
CV 6
CV 4
HP 6
H 6
H 7
St 36
St 37
St 43
Liv 3
Liv 2
St 44

Tai yang
Bitong
LI 20
TH 17
SI 19
GB 12
GB 20
TH 6
TH 5
LI 4
B 54
GB 34
B 57
GB 37
Sp 6
K 6
Sp 4
Sp 1

KEY

B	Bladder
CV	Conception Vessel
GB	Gallbladder
GV	Governing Vessel
H	Heart
HP	Heart Protector
K	Kidney
Liv	Liver
LI	Large Intestine
SI	Small Intestine
Sp	Spleen
St	Stomach
TH	Triple Heater

"read" your body, finding out more about the flow of energy and how it is affecting your health. Most people feel both refreshed and relaxed at the end of such a session. However, occasionally a person may feel slightly worse before feeling better, with fatigue, headaches, or flu-like symptoms. These symptoms, thought to be caused by the release of pent-up energy from the acupressure points, should not be severe or last longer than one or two days.

Using the therapy at home

Self-treatment with acupressure may provide relief from a variety of common ailments, but you can undertake a much wider range of treatments with the help of a partner.

To use acupressure effectively, you first need to find the required pressure point by carefully following the instructions given for the specific ailment. Then apply the correct type of pressure

---

Special precautions

Acupressure is generally safe, provided that the person who is giving the treatment is not too forceful. Do not use acupressure directly over inflamed, swollen, very tender, or recently injured areas; treat only points above or below such areas, or points on the opposite side of the body. Always consult your doctor first if you have a high fever or severe pain, if you have had an accident or injury and suspect that there might be broken bones or concussion, or if you are unsure of the cause of your symptoms.

Pregnancy
With a pregnant woman, avoid strong downward pressure anywhere along the tops of the shoulders. The following acupressure points must not be treated during pregnancy, since it is believed that doing so may cause miscarriage:
- The point (LI 4) in the web between the thumb and index finger on the back of the hand.
- The point (Sp 6) four finger-widths above the inside ankle bone, just behind the tibia.
- All bladder (B) points below the chest and upper back (see p. 25).

Children and the elderly
Be careful if treating a child or an elderly person. The bones may be somewhat fragile, so press gently on points.

The right touch
The thumb is the perfect tool for acupressure. Use the rest of the hand to steady your thumb as you press.

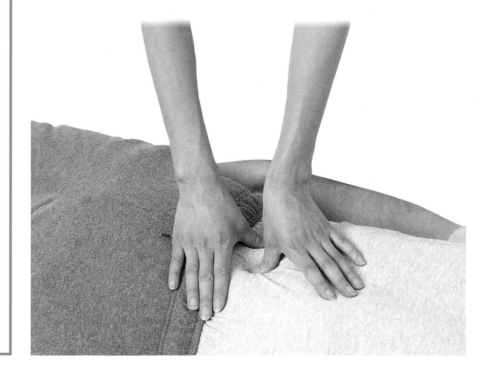

to the point. By using acupressure on yourself, you will learn what it feels like and how to provide the right amount of pressure. If you are ill, certain points may become tender, and pressure may make the point hurt a bit. However, any slight pain should ease after a few moments if you stay relaxed during your treatment. If a minor ailment is not better within two or three days following acupressure, or if your condition seems serious or worsens, consult your doctor.

Treatment by a partner

Lie on a blanket or a rug on the floor. Do not start until you feel comfortable—your treatments will be more effective if you are relaxed. Your partner should sit or kneel by your side and lean towards you, using his or her weight to apply gentle pressure to the appropriate points. The instructions that follow are for your partner.

Thumb technique: Use the pad of your thumb, which you should keep straight. Rest your extended fingers on an adjacent part of the person's body to give you support as you press.

■ Feel for the pressure point, which is a hollow under the skin. Once you feel the bottom of the hollow, release your pressure slightly; this will encourage the qi to respond.

■ Press firmly, but do not use too much force.

■ Use the rhythm of your breathing to time the treatment. As you press, count two or three breaths before gently releasing and then repeating the pressure for two or three more breaths.

■ Press and release several times for each point, remaining aware of your own breath to help you maintain the rhythm and to keep relaxed.

Self-treatment techniques

If you are treating yourself, sit in an upright chair or on pillows. Do not start until you feel comfortable, and make especially sure that the part of the body you are working on is well supported and relaxed. Do not lean your head too close to the area on which you are working. Work at arm's length, with your thumb held straight, so that it feels like an extension of your arm. To work on your arm, rest the hand of that arm on your lap. If you are working on your head or face, practise letting the weight of your head relax down onto your fingertips rather than applying pressure upward or inward with your arm. It may help to rest your elbows on a table when you are treating yourself in this way.

Types of pressure: You can use three types of pressure, to regulate the flow of energy in different ways. "Tonifying" stimulates a weak flow of energy; "dispersing" releases blocked energy, restoring the flow along the meridian; "calming" slows down the flow of overactive energy.

■ To tonify, keep your thumb stationary as you press, and hold the pressure steadily for about two minutes.

■ To disperse energy, move your thumb in a circular motion as you press. Continue for about two minutes.

■ For a calming effect, cover the point with your palm or stroke the point gently for about two minutes.

Aromatherapy

Every plant contains a unique combination of oils in its roots, stems, leaves, seeds, and flowers, which is known as its essential oil. The essential oils of selected plants are used in aromatherapy to foster balance and harmony of the body, mind, and spirit. It is thought that the therapeutic benefit of these oils may result from their effect on hormones and other chemical messengers in the body and brain.

The use of essential oils goes back to at least 4500 B.C., when the Egyptians created perfumes and medicines from them. The Egyptians linked perfumery to religion, assigning a particular fragrance to each of their many deities. Their priests also included essential oils in the embalming process, and traces of these substances can still be detected on 3,000-year-old mummies.

This ancient knowledge was preserved by Greek, Roman, and Arab doctors, whose work was influential for centuries. Even as recently as the 18th century, essential oils were widely used in medicines. But by the late 19th century, many of these extracts could be produced synthetically. This was a cheaper, easier process than obtaining these substances from plants, and the use of natural medicines began to decline.

Modern aromatherapy began with the work of the French chemist René-Maurice Gattefossé, who discovered the healing properties of lavender oil in the 1920s. This encouraged him to investigate the antiseptic properties of essential oils, and in 1937 he published the first modern book on aromatherapy.

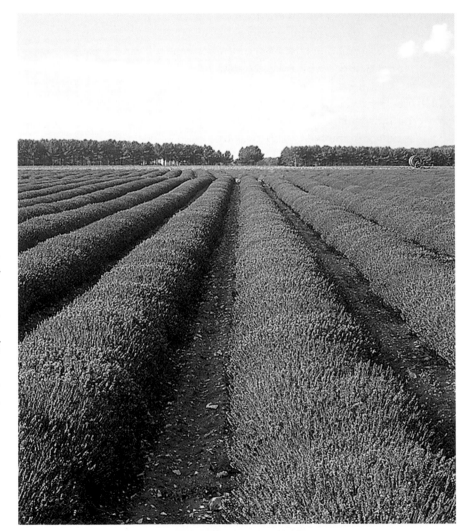

Fields of flowers
Lavender (right), which contains the first essential oil to be investigated in modern times, is grown abundantly in the south of France.

Consulting a professional

An aromatherapist will begin by asking you about your health, your stress levels, and your current mood. There will also be questions about any other remedies you are taking, since the action of certain medicines, especially homeopathic treatments, may be affected by the powerful smell of many aromatherapy oils.

When the aromatherapist has chosen the best oils for you, he or she will decide how to administer the treatment. There are several ways in which a professional therapist can do this, but the most common form of treatment is to give a relaxing, full-body massage with the oils.

After the massage, you will have some time to relax quietly. The therapist may advise you not to bathe for several hours after the massage, so that much of the oil is absorbed into your body. You may be given some oils for home use. The full session, including both consultation and massage, will probably last between 60 and 90 minutes.

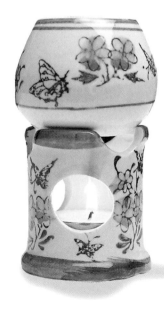

Relaxing fragrance
A vaporizer releases essential oils into the atmosphere. Place a few drops of oil in the water-filled top section and light the candle beneath (don't leave unattended).

Basic mixing of lotions and oils

Before using an essential oil for massage or bathing, you should dilute the oil in a suitable substance, known as a carrier. For massage, use a good quality, cold-pressed plant oil, such as sweet almond, grapeseed, or sunflower oil, as a carrier. For bathing, mix the oils in an unscented white lotion or bubble bath base and then add the mixture to the water. Mix the oils and carrier in the proportions shown below. Do not add more than the specified amount of essential oil; it will not increase the benefit.

Standard mix for bathing	30 drops of essential oil in 20 teaspoons of carrier
Bathing mix for the young, elderly, and those in poor health	16 drops of essential oil in 20 teaspoons of carrier
Bathing mix for babies under 2 years old	8 drops of essential oil in 20 teaspoons of carrier
Massage oil	8–12 drops of essential oil in 6–8 teaspoons of carrier

---

Using this therapy at home

It is important to obtain a reliable medical diagnosis before using aromatherapy to treat symptoms for which you would normally consult your doctor. Essential oils are widely available, and such treatments as inhalation, massage, and bathing are simple to carry out at home. But the oils will be effective only if they have been extracted carefully and stored correctly.

The best oils are sold in dark-glass bottles with labels showing the Latin name of the plant, instructions for use, and precautions listed clearly. Quality oils are usually labelled "true" or "pure" essential oil, and are produced by steam distillation or expression from natural, usually organically grown, plant material.

Special precautions

Although pure essential oils can help skin problems and can be absorbed into the bloodstream to spread their benefits around the body, some synthetic oils may cause skin reactions or trigger asthma attacks. Use the purest essential oils available to ensure you receive the maximum benefit and to reduce the risks.

If you have sensitive skin, epilepsy, high blood pressure, or have recently had an operation, you should consult a qualified practitioner before using essential oils to check whether they are safe to use.

If you are or might be pregnant, you should avoid certain essential oils, such as those listed below. If in doubt, consult a qualified aromatherapist.

Oils to avoid in the first 20 weeks of pregnancy

- Basil *(Ocimum basilicum)*
- Cajuput *(Melaleuca leucadendron)*
- Cedarwood *(Cedrus atlantica)*
- Clary sage *(Salvia sclarea)*
- Cypress *(Cupressus sempervirens)*
- Myrrh *(Commiphora myrrha)*
- Niaouli *(Melaleuca viridiflora)*
- Rosemary *(Rosmarinus officinalis)*

Oils to avoid throughout pregnancy

- Angelica *(Angelica archangelica)*
- Aniseed *(Pimpinella anisum)*
- Camphor *(Cinnamomum camphora)*
- Caraway *(Carum carvi)*
- Clove *(Eugenia caryophyllata)*
- Cinnamon *(Cinnamomum zeylanicum)*
- Fennel *(Foeniculum vulgare)*
- Hyssop *(Hyssopus officinalis)*
- Juniper berry *(Juniperus communis)*
- Lemongrass *(Cymbopogon citratus)*
- Nutmeg *(Myristica fragrans)*
- Oregano *(Origanum vulgare)*
- Parsley *(Petroselinum crispum)*
- Pennyroyal *(Mentha pulegium)*
- Savory *(Satureia montana)*
- Tarragon *(Artemisia dracunculus)*
- Thyme, red *(Thymus vulgaris, chemotype—or ct—thymol or carvacrol)*

Buy from a reputable source (ask an aromatherapist for advice) and keep your oils in a cool place in tightly sealed, dark-glass bottles. Choose the oils you need by listing those that are effective for your particular ailments and then selecting the most appropriate. Before using an essential oil for massage or bathing, you should dilute it in a suitable substance, known as a carrier (see box, page 29). Mix the oils and carrier oil or lotion in the proportions recommended. You can prepare enough for several uses in advance. If the oil or blend of oils you have chosen does not improve your condition, consider consulting a suitably qualified therapist for advice.

Inhaling: This is the quickest way to get an essential oil into the bloodstream. There are two simple ways of inhaling oils:

- Place a few drops of the volatile oil on a tissue, put the tissue to your nose, and inhale.
- Add one or two drops of essential oil to a bowl of hot water, place a towel around your head and over the bowl, and inhale the vapour for up to five minutes.

You can repeat either treatment up to three times daily, as required. Or use your chosen oils in a vaporizer (see photograph, p. 29). Be aware, however, that this method provides a less concentrated dose and is therefore more suitable for mild mood-lifting or soothing effects.

Bathing: Soaking in water to which you have added essential oils is one of the simplest ways of absorbing oils into your body.

- Use about 10 teaspoons of carrier to which you have added essential oils in the proportions recommended in the box on page 29. (If you add oils to a bath without a carrier, they will float on the top of the water and the therapeutic benefits may be reduced.)
- Swirl the water around so that the oil disperses.
- Close the door and windows and relax in the bath for 10 minutes.

Popular aromatherapy oils

Oil	Possible benefits: mental	Possible benefits: physical
Eucalyptus *Eucalyptus globulus*	Promotes alertness; clears the mind	Helps fight colds and congestion; soothes dry coughs; combats skin infections, such as boils and pimples; reduces swellings and muscle aches and pains
Geranium *Pelargonium graveolens*	Helps reduce mental stress and anxiety	Tones and cleanses the skin; fights throat and mouth infections; stimulates the liver and cleanses the digestive system; helps the body remove waste products; combats fluid retention
Lavender *Lavandula officinalis*	Combats anxiety, stress, and depression	Stimulates renewal of skin cells; reduces skin inflammation; helps heal mouth ulcers; reduces bad breath and nausea
Peppermint *Mentha piperita*	Uplifting; useful in treatment of emotional shock	Helps reduce coughs and throat infections; soothes intestinal cramps and heartburn; alleviates motion sickness
Roman chamomile *Chamaemelum nobile*	Relaxing; reduces anxiety; often effective for calming children's tantrums	Helps clear acne, rashes, and skin inflammation; reduces muscle inflammation; stimulates appetite; combats diarrhoea
Rosemary *Rosmarinus officinalis*	Stimulates the memory	Relieves indigestion and flatulence; helps circulation; alleviates muscular aches; cleanses and stimulates the skin; counters infection
Sandalwood *Santalum album*	Sedative and relaxing; good remedy for insomnia	Soothes throat irritation, bronchitis, and asthma; softens dry skin; combats dandruff; alleviates vomiting and diarrhoea
Sweet marjoram *Origanum marjorana*	Calms and comforts in cases of grief, loneliness, and loss	Eases respiratory problems, such as bronchitis and asthma; helps relieve constipation; relaxes muscle cramps
Tea tree *Melaleuca alternifolia*	No special benefits	Works as antiseptic against bacterial infections, particularly of the skin; used for cleaning cuts and surface wounds

Flower Essences

Made from the blossoms of plants and trees, flower essences are first prepared in water and then preserved in alcohol. They are used for their possible therapeutic impact on the mind and the spirit, and it is believed that they may help to reverse negative mental states and rebalance the emotions. Their gentle action—there are no known adverse effects—makes them an ideal complement to other treatments.

The first person to prepare flower essences was Dr. Edward Bach, a bacteriologist and pathologist working in Wales in the 1930s. Bach became convinced that human illnesses were often symptoms of basic imbalances in the personality and the emotional life. He believed that flowers had the power to ease mental stress, and he used intuition and self-testing to investigate the therapeutic effects of a variety of flowers. To begin with, he prepared a dozen flower essences and called them the "Twelve Healers" (see facing page). These were followed by another 26 remedies, making a total of 38. Each essence is said to help dissipate a particular unpleasant emotion, such as fear, impatience, or worry. Bach prepared his remedies as liquids so that they would be easy to mix together to create personalized treatments. In recent decades, people all over the world have borrowed Bach's ideas to make new flower-based preparations, adding to the number of essences and combination remedies available for use.

Consulting a professional

A practitioner will draw upon two kinds of flower essences to arrive at a personalized mix for a client. Those that describe someone's personality are known as "type" essences, while those that describe a mood are called "mood" or "helper" essences. The practitioner usually prescribes a blend that includes both kinds of essences. For example, a normally authoritarian person who is anxious about having to make a speech at a wedding might be given Vine as a type essence and Mimulus as a helper for his fear. Simple problems may require only one essence.

Flower-essence practitioners do not delve too deeply into the underlying causes of psychological states. Instead, troublesome emotions that have accumulated over years are resolved slowly, layer by layer. Most practitioners stick to what is

Healing holly
The flower essence which is derived from the holly bush is said to counteract envy and hatred.

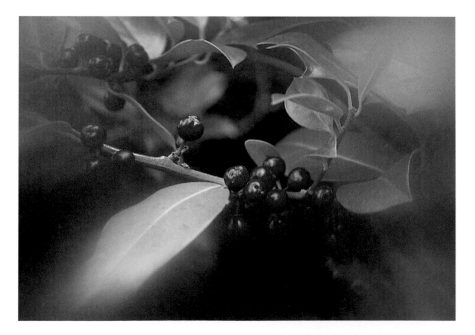

An all-purpose elixir

Dr. Edward Bach called his most famous flower essence Rescue Remedy. This is a mix of five different essences selected to help people through crises and emergencies of all kinds. Take four drops in a glass of water, or put the drops straight onto your tongue if no water is readily available.

on the surface and give the essences time to work on a person's most obvious problems as they arise. Always seek your doctor's advice about any worrying symptoms. More than most other therapies, flower essences are meant to be a complementary treatment. They do not take the place of conventional care for medical conditions, but rather are intended to help you deal with underlying emotional problems that may have caused or are complicating your condition.

Using this therapy at home

You can experiment with flower essences secure in the knowledge that selecting the wrong essence will not do you any harm. If you feel stuck, or if you have taken your own carefully selected essences for three weeks with no improvement, consult a professional.

When selecting flower essences for yourself, take the time to think about how you feel, and match your feelings to the essences. You can take up to seven essences at one time. If you intend to use flower essences on a regular basis, consider investing in a reference book that gives full details about each remedy.

Making a personal mixture

- Put two drops of each of your chosen essences into an empty one-fluid-ounce dropper bottle.
- Add a teaspoon of brandy and then fill to the top of the bottle with still mineral water. Use glycerine instead of brandy if you prefer to avoid alcohol.
- Take four drops four times a day, or more frequently if you feel the need.
- The treatment bottle will last two to three weeks if you take the essence regularly. When you have used it up, take a fresh look at your emotions. If you need to, make up another bottle with the same or different essences.
- For passing moods, simply add two drops of the essences you need to a glass of water, or drop each essence directly onto your tongue.

Special precautions

Flower essences are safe—even for babies and pregnant women. However, alcohol is generally used to preserve them. If this may be a problem, make your own with glycerine instead of alcohol or consult a qualified practitioner. The essences do not react with other medicines.

The Twelve Healers

Essence	Principal symptoms
Agrimony	Concealed anxiety
Centaury	Excessive desire to please, lack of assertiveness
Cerato	Doubting your own judgment and decision-making
Chicory	Excessive interference in the concerns of others
Clematis	Absent-mindedness, dreaminess
Gentian	Despondency
Impatiens	Impatience
Mimulus	Shyness, anxiety, everyday fears
Rock Rose	Terror
Scleranthus	Indecision, mood swings
Vervain	Extremes of energy and enthusiasm
Water Violet	Excessive self-sufficiency, aloofness

Herbal Medicine

The use of plant remedies to strengthen weakened body systems, control symptoms, and boost the body's own healing powers is perhaps the oldest form of medicine. Herbalists maintain that the natural balance of compounds in plants provides a more effective means of dealing with imbalances within the body and restoring health than the synthesized, single ingredient drugs which are prescribed in orthodox modern medicine.

No one knows how or when people realized that plants could be used to treat disease, but herbal medicine probably developed from the use of plants as foods, partly by a system of trial and error, and partly from knowledge gained by people living close to nature that has been handed down through the generations.

With the development of science, it became possible to isolate plant compounds and to find out which chemicals in a plant have particular actions. These chemicals were duplicated in laboratories to produce what we now call orthodox medicines. The work undertaken by medical researchers has given herbalists a wider understanding of why herbs have particular effects on the body. But this insight has not changed the way herbalists work.

Herbalists have always believed, and continue to believe, that using whole plants, which contain a huge variety of compounds, is the ideal way to help strengthen the body's healing powers and to help restore any imbalances in the body. Although a plant may be chosen primarily for the action of one ingredient, the other compounds in the plant—or in several plants in a combination remedy—may limit or enhance the main action, prevent side effects, or act in a generally nutritive way. Some herbal products contain several active compounds in an extract from the whole plant. Others contain only one or two compounds that have been isolated from the plant. A standardized extract contains known amounts of one or more active compounds.

Consulting a professional

Herbal remedies can be used to treat many common ailments, as well as to enhance energy

---

Buying and using herbs safely

- Ensure your ailment is diagnosed correctly before using herbal medicine.
- Use only herbs specifically recommended in this book or by a doctor.
- Tell your doctor about any herbs you plan to take.
- Buy herbs from a well-established company. Choose a brand with an address and telephone number on the packaging, so that you can ask questions about the herb.
- Be aware that manufacturers of herbal remedies in the UK can make therapeutic claims on the product's packaging only if the remedy is a licensed medicine. However, most remedies are unlicensed. The Medicines Control Agency is working with herbal interest groups to improve regulations about consumer information.
- Avoid bulk herbs (sold loose) that may have been exposed to light and air for long periods.
- Choose products with evidence of quality control testing, especially the herbs standardized for one or more of the active ingredients.
- Be aware that herbal tinctures are often prepared in a base of water and alcohol. If you want to avoid alcohol, buy tinctures in a glycerine base.
- Bear in mind the shelf lives of different forms of herbs. Bulk herbs can last from three months (for leaves and flowers) to a year (for roots and bark); tinctures about a year; capsules and tablets one to two years.
- If you are interested in using herbal remedies on a regular basis, invest in a sound reference book that gives full information about specific herbs.

Special precautions

- Herbal remedies contain active constituents that can be harmful if taken in excess. Keep to recommended strengths and doses, and if in any doubt, consult a doctor familiar with herbal medicines.
- With remedies bought over the counter, keep to the dose recommended on the label.
- Do not take herbal remedies in combination with orthodox medicines without the approval of your doctor.
- Always check with your doctor before taking herbal medicines if you are or might be pregnant or you are breastfeeding, if you have any medical condition, or if you are over 70 and in poor health.
- Do not give herbal medicines to children under 16 without first checking with your doctor. Expert advice is needed to determine the correct dosage.

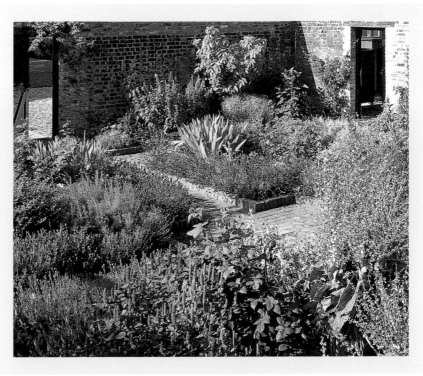

A healing garden
In times gone by, many hospitals, often run by religious orders, maintained their own herb gardens to ensure a constant supply of herbal medicines.

and immunity. Athough they are suitable for self-treatment, it is often best to seek advice from a professional practitioner of herbal medicine (see "Special precautions", above). Some fully qualified doctors have also studied herbal medicine. Naturopaths are not usually medically qualified, but have undergone extensive training. You should ensure that any practitioner you consult has qualifications from the National Institute of Medical Herbalists.

When you visit a herbalist, he or she will ask about your medical history, paying especially close attention to your diet and lifestyle. If neces-sary, the therapist will perform a physical examination. Having assessed your condition, the herbalist then looks for the root cause of the problem, trying to find out where any imbalance in your health could have occurred. The practitioner believes that until this is addressed, the underlying problem will not be resolved, although it may be possible to alleviate or suppress the symptoms.

The herbalist will give dietary advice, suggesting changes that may help the patient better deal with the stresses of life. He or she may then recommend a blend of herbal remedies

Strain well
Use a fine strainer to remove the coarse, woody pieces of plant material that remain after you have simmered a herb for a decoction.

specially suited to your individual needs. The initial consultation usually takes about one hour. Subsequent sessions, when the herbalist may suggest adjustments, take about half an hour.

Using this therapy at home

Medicinal herbs lend themselves well to home use, and many of them are easy and fun to grow in your garden or window box. However, it is important to recognize that they *are* medicines —some can be taken safely in large amounts; others cannot. It is also very important to be certain, if collecting herbs yourself, that you collect the right plants. The best way is to learn this from an expert. Never consume a herb unless you are absolutely sure that you have identified it correctly.

Herbal remedies should generally be taken until symptoms disappear. If this does not happen within two weeks, if the condition worsens, or if any unexpected effects occur, stop taking the preparation and seek medical help.

Taking herbs by mouth

Many herbs are available from health-food stores as tablets, capsules, or tinctures (extracts in alcohol). Follow the dosage instructions on the package, starting with the lowest dose.

The traditional way to take herbs by mouth is in the form of teas. There are two kinds of herbal tea. The type of tea made with the flowers or leaves of a plant is called an infusion. It is made by pouring boiling water over the herb to release the active ingredients. The hard or woody parts of a herb, such as the roots, bark, seeds, or berries, need to be simmered in water for some time to bring out the healing constituents. This is known as a decoction. In Part Two of this book, the term *tea* has been used to describe both forms of preparation. Herbal teas may be drunk hot or cold.

Dosages for teas vary according to your age and health, but the usual amount for adults is one cup three times a day. Elderly people should take half this dose. Seek professional advice before giving herbs to children under 16 years old.

How to make an infusion: This type of herbal preparation is made rather like ordinary tea. You can make either a whole pot to provide several doses, or a single cup for one dose.
- To make a pot, pour one pint of boiling water over one ounce of dried herb (or two ounces of fresh). Cover, and leave to infuse for 5 to 10 minutes. Strain, and pour into a cup.
- To make a single cup, put one teaspoon of dried herb (or two teaspoons of fresh) into a cup, pour on boiling water, and leave covered for five minutes. Strain, then use.

How to make a decoction: This type of herbal preparation is made by simmering hard plant material over low heat.
- Gently simmer one ounce of the herb in one pint of water for at least 15 minutes.
- Strain to remove the plant material.
- Some of the liquid will have evaporated, so add more water until you have one pint again.

Using herbs externally

You can buy a wide variety of herbal creams, lotions, and other products for external use. These can be convenient when you need a remedy for immediate use, as for first aid. However, preparing your own can give greater control over the ingredients. Some herbal applications are not available commercially.

Herbal baths: These provide an easy and pleasant way of gaining benefit from herbs.
- Hang a calico bag containing the chosen dried or fresh herbs under the hot tap when running the bath.
- Prepare a herbal hand or foot bath by adding a strong infusion or decoction of the herb(s) to a bowl of hot water. Soak your hands or feet in the mixture until the water cools.

Steam inhalations: You can use fresh or dried herbs. Make a strong infusion of the herb in a ceramic or glass bowl. Place your face over the bowl with a towel over your head, and breathe in the steam.

Compresses: Herbal compresses are helpful in the treatment of sprains and bruises, to cool fevers or inflammation, and to soothe headaches.
- Soak a clean cloth in a strong infusion or decoction (used hot or cold as recommended), or in a diluted tincture.
- After wringing excess liquid from the cloth, wrap it around the affected area.
- Repeat as necessary.

Poultices: Commonly used to draw pus from ulcers or boils, herbal poultices can also ease nerve or muscle pain. Make a poultice from fresh or dried herbs.
- Chop the herbs finely, cover with water, and heat to boiling.
- Put the resultant paste of hot herbs between two pieces of gauze, and apply to the affected area while still hot.
- Secure the poultice (see photograph, right).
- Use a hot-water bottle to keep the poultice warm.
- Replace the poultice when it has cooled.

Kept in place
Bind a herbal poultice to the affected area with a cotton bandage secured with tape or a safety pin.

Homeopathy

The word homeopathy is derived from the Greek words *omeo pathos*, which means "similar suffering". The therapy is based on the principle that "like cures like". Homeopaths believe that if a substance can produce the symptoms of illness when taken in a large dose, it has the potential to heal the same symptoms when taken in an infinitesimally small dose. And this treatment can be applied without causing any harm to the patient.

The concept of "like curing like" has been around for thousands of years, but the development of homeopathy as a medical system took place only relatively recently, with the work of the German doctor, chemist, and linguist Samuel Hahnemann (1755–1843).

With homeopathy, Hahnemann developed a system that embraces a natural form of healing which treats the whole person, not just the symptoms of illness. He "proved", or tested, about 100 remedies, almost all of which are regularly used today. Many more remedies have been discovered since Hahnemann's time. Remedies are prepared from many sources (plants, minerals, even venoms) but are given in such small amounts that they are gentle and safe. The full name of a homeopathic remedy is usually the Latin for the plant or other source material, for example, *Arsenicum album*. However, most homeopaths use abbreviated forms, either the first word of the Latin name (the form used in this book)—in this example, Arsenicum—or a shortened form of both words—Ars. alb.

Consulting a professional

The first time you visit a qualified practitioner, he or she will ask you about your medical history, lifestyle, diet, likes, dislikes, and personality, as well as your illness, to help determine your physical and emotional type. Hardly any physical examination is needed because the key to an accurate homeopathic diagnosis is listening and understanding.

Homeopaths believe that, as a rule, people are self-healing, provided that they are properly fed and cared for. So a homeopath treats symptoms of illness as signs that the body is fighting disease, and he or she will prescribe a remedy that, in a larger dose, would produce similar symptoms. The purpose of homeopathic treatment is to stimulate your powers of self-healing. The practitioner therefore usually seeks a remedy that suits you as a whole person, rather than one that simply addresses your symptoms. Generally, only one remedy at a time will be prescribed. Shorter return appointments, often three or four weeks apart, are usually necessary.

Taking the remedy
Handle only the pill you are taking. You may find it easier to shake the pill onto a spoon first.

It is advisable to seek out an expert practitioner if you have a long-term disease, if you are very worried by your illness, or if you have tried several remedies without success—all of these circumstances also necessitate seeing a medical doctor. When treating children or the elderly, it is a good idea to consult a professional first.

Using the therapy at home

Always obtain a medical diagnosis for symptoms for which you would normally seek your doctor's advice before attempting home treatment. Most homeopathic remedies are readily available, usually in the form of pills. For injuries, a topical cream, which you apply liberally and rub in gently, may be used. Choose homeopathic calen-

dula (marigold) cream for minor cuts and sores, and Hypercal cream for insect bites.

Throughout this book, you will find instructions on which remedies to use for particular ailments. But you should always bear in mind that, when prescribing, homeopaths take into account not only your symptoms but also your mood, personality, and constitutional type.

Taking homeopathic pills: The pills are sweet because they contain milk sugar (lactose).
■ Dosage intervals vary from once an hour to once a day, according to your condition.
■ Take the pills on a clean tongue, preferably allowing a 15-minute gap after meals or after cleaning your teeth.
■ Some practitioners recommend that you avoid caffeine while you are having homeopathic treatments, as it may reduce their effectiveness.
■ Suck the pill for about 30 seconds before chewing and swallowing.
■ When your symptoms begin to subside, stop taking the remedy. If they return, start again. If there is no improvement in an acute illness within 24 hours, choose another remedy.

Constitutional remedies

When you visit a professional homeopath, he or she may seem just as interested in your medical history, character, and likes and dislikes as in your current illness. This is because the practitioner is trying to build up a picture of your whole nature, or constitution. He or she may then try to find a remedy that suits your constitution, rather than just your specific ailment. A constitutional remedy is often considered especially effective for a chronic condition, such as arthritis.

Less is more

Turning a substance into a homeopathic remedy is a process called potentization. This involves alternately diluting and shaking the substance, often until no physical molecules of the original substance remain. Homeopaths believe that the more times this is carried out, the more powerful the remedy becomes. In other words, the more dilute the solution, the stronger its effect. Remedies are normally given a number and a letter—for example, 30c. This means that the process of diluting and shaking has been carried out 30 times, starting with a dilution of one part in 100 each time. For home use, the sixth potency (6c) is ideal.

Special precautions

Because homeopathic remedies are used in such minute dilutions, there is little chance of any harm arising from overprescribing. However, a remedy may cause a temporary worsening of symptoms before it starts to relieve them. Remedies from the sixth (6c) to thirtieth (30c) potency are safe for people of all ages, including pregnant women. For babies and young children, crush each pill to a fine powder.

39

Common homeopathic remedies

This chart correlates symptoms with 18 of the most widely used homeopathic remedies (with alternative abbreviated names in brackets). Refer to the appropriate article in Part Two of this book for advice on treating specific ailments.

Remedy	Origin	Symptoms
Aconite	The monkshood plant, *Aconitum napellus*	High fever, often coming suddenly in the night; extreme thirst and perspiration; symptoms that may arise from a chill or fright; dry coughs in children; fear or extreme anxiety along with other symptoms
Apis	The honeybee, *Apis mellifica*	Swelling in which the affected area is red and puffy or seems fluid-filled; burning and stinging pains; irritability and restlessness; symptoms that are relieved by cool air or cold compresses
Arnica	A perennial herb of mountainous regions, *Arnica montana*	Shock from injury; muscle strain, jet lag, post-operative recovery
Arsenicum album (Ars. alb.)	Arsenic trioxide, a poisonous white powder that is safe in homeopathic doses	Vomiting, diarrhoea, abdominal and stomach cramps, such as might arise after food poisoning; head colds with runny nose; symptoms relieved by warmth and sips of cold water; anxiety, chilliness, restlessness, and weakness along with symptoms
Belladonna	The deadly nightshade plant, *Atropa belladonna*	High fever, perhaps with delirium, which comes on suddenly; burning dry skin, red face, and little thirst with the fever; throbbing pains, especially in the head area; dilated pupils and oversensitivity to light
Bryonia (Bry.)	The bryony plant, *Bryonia alba*	Slowly developing fever; dry, painful coughs relieved by holding the chest; extreme thirst for large amounts of cold water; symptoms that are worse for slight motion; irritability, desire to be left alone
Chamomilla (Cham.)	German or wild chamomile, *Matricaria chamomilla*	Any illness, especially in children, that includes bad temper and irritability; teething and colic, with irritability
Gelsemium (Gels.)	The yellow jasmine of North America, *Gelsemium sempervirens*	Flu—with weak, achy muscles, tiredness, weakness, shivering, fever, little thirst; anxiety that includes trembling

Remedy	Origin	Symptoms
Hepar sulphuris calcareum (Hepar sulph.)	A compound of calcium and sulphur made by heating oyster shells and calcium sulphide together	Sore throat that feels as though something is stuck in your throat; harsh, dry cough with yellow mucus; boils and abscesses that will not heal; extreme irritability, coldness, and sour-smelling perspiration
Hypericum (Hyper.)	The European herb St. John's wort, *Hypericum perforatum*	Bruising of very sensitive areas, such as fingers, toes, lips, ears, eyes, and coccyx; shooting pains along nerve pathways
Ignatia (Ign.)	St. Ignatius' bean, a tree that grows in China	Sadness and grief following emotional loss; "locked-up" grief, in which the tears will not flow; mood swings
Ipecacuanha (Ipecac.)	The dried root of the South American shrub, *Cephaëlis ipecacuanha*	Nausea and vomiting, whether or not accompanied by other symptoms, such as coughing, wheezing, headache, or diarrhoea; morning sickness
Ledum (Led.)	The small shrub known as marsh tea, *Ledum palustre*	Puncture wounds, as from splinters, nails, or stings, that look puffy and feel cold; pain eased by cold compresses; eye injuries that look puffy and bloodshot and that feel cold to touch
Mercurius (Merc.)	The metal mercury	Swollen lymph nodes ("glands"), coated tongue, profuse sweating, increased thirst; offensive breath and perspiration; feeling alternately hot and cold; irritability and restlessness along with other symptoms
Nux vomica (Nux vom.)	The poison nut tree, *Strychnos nux vomica,* native to eastern Asia	Gastrointestinal upset, especially after a rich meal; undigested food lying like a weight in the stomach; feeling of nausea, but inability to vomit; feeling that bowel movements are incomplete; heartburn
Pulsatilla (Puls.)	The pasqueflower *Pulsatilla nigricans,* a member of the anemone family	Conditions in which emotional symptoms such as weepiness, clinginess, and changeable moods predominate, especially in children; yellow-green discharges, as from nose or eyes; menstrual problems; symptoms that are helped by sympathy and hugs, as well as fresh, cool air
Rhus toxico-dendron (Rhus tox.)	The North American poison ivy	Sprains and stiffness in the joints that are eased by gentle motion; symptoms that are better for warmth and worse for cold and damp, or are accompanied by extreme restlessness; red, itchy, painful rashes
Ruta	The herb rue, *Ruta graveolens*	Bruises near the bones, as from a kick on the shin; strains to joints, especially ankles and wrists; symptoms that are better for warmth and worse for cold and damp; eyestrain from overwork

Massage

The use of touch to promote a sense of physical and emotional well-being is one of the oldest of all natural therapies. Massage employs many different strokes that can stimulate or relax muscles, improve circulation, and encourage healing of a wide variety of complaints. This therapy can also be used in conjunction with aromatherapy, as massaging essential oils or lotions into the skin can achieve a broad range of therapeutic benefits.

Touch is one of the most basic of the senses, experienced even by babies still in the uterus. Chinese physicians have made use of this knowledge for thousands of years. In China, massage is part of the system of traditional medicine that also includes acupuncture. The doctors of ancient Greece and Rome used massage, but the therapy disappeared from the West in the Middle Ages. Massage became popular again largely due to the work of a Swede, Per Henrik Ling, who developed Swedish movement treatment, or Swedish massage, in the early part of the 19th century.

During the 20th century, many types of massage have developed. Some derive from Ling's work; others are influenced by Chinese and Japanese medicine. They are all beneficial to the muscular system, relaxing tight muscles and toning loose ones. There are, in addition, more wide-reaching effects, because massage helps the circulation of the blood and lymph.

According to Chinese practitioners, massage also promotes the flow of vital energy, or *qi*, along a network of channels, or meridians, to all parts of the body, and so can be used in the treatment of many ailments. One specialized therapy, shiatsu, is based on a form of massage developed in Japan that works specifically on points where meridians (or energy channels) are thought to be near the surface of the skin. This is believed to regulate the flow of energy (see p. 24).

Consulting a professional

When you book a professional massage, you will probably be advised to avoid drinking alcohol on the day of the appointment and to abstain from eating for about two hours before the massage.

The massage itself will vary according to your problem. The therapist may concentrate on one area or work on your whole body. The treatment should not be painful, although stiff muscles may feel uncomfortable during massage. At the end of the session, the therapist may "ground" you by holding your feet for 20 seconds or so. You will then be given some time on your own to lie still.

After the massage, you may feel either relaxed or full of energy. Your muscles may be a little stiff for a while afterwards, especially if they had previously been causing you pain. If muscle stiffness is likely, the therapist may advise you to lie for 30 minutes in a warm bath when you get home. Towel yourself down briskly afterwards.

➤ continued, p. 45

A healing experience
An effective massage (right) depends on the sense of ease created by comfortable surroundings and trust in the masseur, as well as the technical expertise with which the strokes are carried out.

Gliding hands
Professional masseurs use a lubricating oil or lotion (left) to help the hands move smoothly across the skin. One who is also familiar with aromatherapy will choose a blend of essential oils that is appropriate for your problem, warming the oil on the hands before rubbing it into your skin.

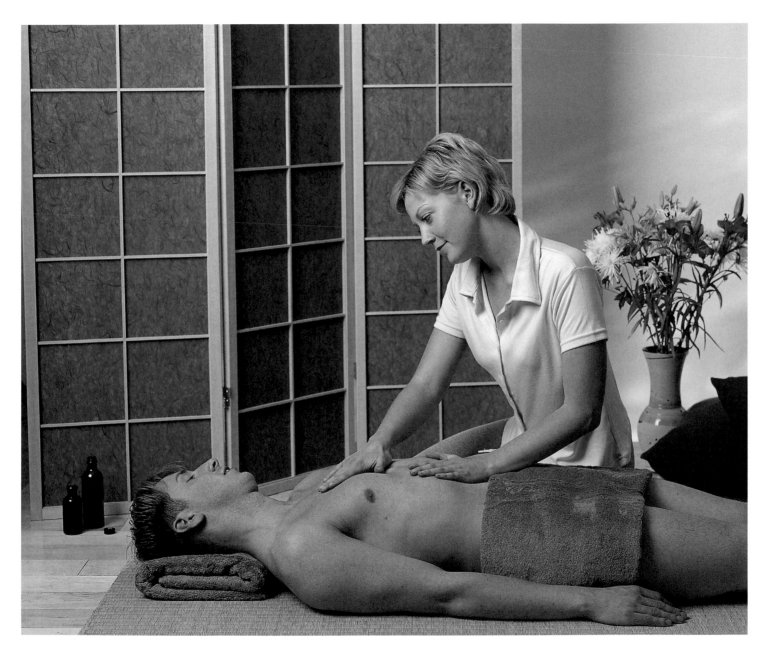

The basic massage strokes

There are three main massage strokes: effleurage, petrissage, and friction. Use these to relax and tone the muscles. (Be sure your fingernails are trimmed before giving a massage.)

Effleurage

This gentle stroke is a good one to use at the beginning of a massage, because it helps you distribute the massage oil across the person's skin. It is a good stroke for general relaxation, but you can also use it for very sore muscles, since it stretches the muscle fibres.

- Hold your hands side by side, with the fingers together; your hands should be relaxed, but not limp.
- Glide your hands along the whole length of the muscles, moving towards the head; on this stroke, keep your palms and fingers in contact with the person's skin, letting your hands feel the contours of the body.
- Make a lighter return stroke, using only your fingertips.

Petrissage

Use this kneading stroke after effleurage. The best places for petrissage are the back, upper chest, legs, and buttocks. The stroke separates tight muscle fibres and helps rid muscles of waste products.

- With your fingers outstretched, put the heels of your hands in the middle of the area on which you are going to work.
- Push with the heel of each hand in turn. Press quite hard, but not so hard that you hurt the person.
- Do not use this stroke for too long on any one area.

Friction

Apply friction massage to a series of specific points or in any place on the back where the muscles are stiff. Use little or no oil; otherwise, you may slip away from the point you are massaging. The main direction of movement should be downwards and circular. Avoid pressing directly on the spine.

- Slowly apply pressure to the point, using the pad of your thumb or index finger. Increase the pressure gradually.
- Rotate very slightly for about 10 to 15 seconds.
- Release the pressure very gradually.
- Repeat once or twice.
- Use effleurage to relax the muscles.

Using the therapy at home

Massage is easy to perform. You can do some types on yourself—for example, on the hands, arms, legs, and shoulders. However, the result is generally better if you perform the massage, following the instructions in this book, on someone else and vice versa.

The only equipment you need to perform a massage is your hands. The kind of massage table used by a professional masseur is helpful, but not essential. The person can either lie on a mattress or the floor and the area should be covered with foam or a thick blanket and a large towel. When you are working on the shoulders, the person should sit on a stool and lean forwards onto the back of an armchair.

Support: Depending on which part of the body you are working on, you may have to provide some additional support.
- If you are massaging someone's back and he or she is lying face down, you should place a pillow under their head and a rolled towel under their knees.
- If you are massaging the calves, support the ankles with a pillow.
- If you are working on the fronts of the legs, place a pillow under their knees.
- If you are massaging the back and shoulders of someone lying face down, put a pillow under the chest.

Oils and lotions: Many different massage oils are available. One of the best for general use is sweet almond oil, but you can also use any cream that is not highly scented and is not absorbed into the skin too quickly. If a person has very oily skin, use powder or cornflour instead of oil, which may make the skin more greasy.

Warmth: Massage is most effective in a relaxed atmosphere, so keep the room warm and quiet. For extra heat and comfort, keep the parts of the body not being massaged covered with a towel.

Pressure: Whichever kind of stroke you are using, this rule applies: the longer the stroke, the lighter it should be, and the shorter the stroke, the deeper it should be. Faster strokes are energizing, slower strokes more sedating. Different people feel comfortable with different levels of pressure, so be guided by the person you are massaging. At the same time, consider your own well-being. Leaning over to give a massage can strain your back, so adopt a comfortable position in which to work and stay as relaxed as you can.

Special precautions
- Do not have a massage if you have a fever.
- If you have recently had surgery, do not have a massage on or near the affected area.
- Do not have a massage if you have just eaten a meal or if you have drunk alcohol on the same day.
- Do not allow massage of bruised or inflamed areas, and avoid pressure on the backs of the knees or on bony areas.
- If you are or might be pregnant, permit only gentle strokes, and do not have massage on the lower back or abdomen. Consider consulting a masseur trained in pregnancy massage.
- If you are undergoing medical treatment, first ask your doctor whether it is safe to have massage.
- If you have unexplained pain, swelling, or illness, consult your doctor before trying a massage.

Meditation

The art of relaxing the mind, known as meditation, is a remarkably simple, straightforward technique. Many people find it easy to fit this therapy into their daily lives and the results are usually very rewarding. In recent years, an increasing number of scientific studies have recognized meditation as a highly effective treatment for a range of problems, both physical and psychological, that can result from stress or a low energy level.

Meditation helps you train your mind to filter out the unwanted distractions of life—the odd worries, concerns, and seemingly random images that spring to mind during the course of our everyday lives. Meditation techniques can induce a serene state, sometimes akin to deep sleep. Mind and body can relax fully, and many people find that just 20 minutes of meditation is as refreshing as several hours of sleep.

People all around the world have been using various forms of meditation for millennia. The ancient yoga practitioners described the practice as a powerful tonic that increases energy, rejuvenates cells, and helps delay signs of aging. Science is now confirming that meditation can be a powerful healer. Researchers have found that it can help reduce the symptoms of high blood pressure, angina, allergies, diabetes, chronic headaches, and bronchial asthma; it can also help reduce dependence on alcohol and cigarettes. Those who meditate see their doctors less and spend fewer days in hospital. Anxiety and depression decrease, while memory improves. Meditation appears to give us more stamina, a happier disposition, and in some cases better relationships.

Joining a meditation class

The easiest way to start meditating is to join a class. There are classes available in all types of meditation. Also, many yoga teachers incorporate meditation into their work, using sound or breathing to focus the mind. You can even learn to chant—a form of sound meditation—choosing from Eastern mantras or Western forms, such as the Gregorian chant developed by medieval monks.

Using meditation at home

Meditation is very simple to practise. Find a quiet, warm place where you will not be disturbed. It is usually best to sit down, adopting whatever position you find comfortable. You may want to sit cross-legged, either directly on the floor or on a firm cushion, three to six inches thick. Or you may prefer to sit in a supportive, straight-backed chair, with your hands resting gently on your knees and your feet flat on the floor. It is not usually a good idea to meditate lying down, because you may fall asleep during the therapy.

Basic meditation exercise: There are many different ways of meditating. Try this basic technique, which suits many people, first. If it does not suit you, consider the variations suggested on the facing page.
- Sit comfortably upright, so that you are alert but not tense.
- Keep your back straight, aligned with your head and neck, and relax your body.

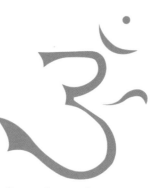

Sacred sound
The Hindu sacred syllable *ohm*, shown above as written in Sanskrit, is often used by practitioners of yoga and other Hindu-based forms of meditation as a "mantra", or sound on which to focus.

- Breathe steadily and deeply. Concentrate on your breath as it flows in and out, and be aware of your abdomen falling and rising. Give your full attention to your breathing.
- If your attention starts to wander, gently bring your thoughts back to your breathing and to the rising and falling of your stomach.
- It is usual to keep eyes gently closed, to help you concentrate.
- Many people find it helpful to repeat a special word or sound, such as *ohm* (see illustration, facing page), the Hebrew word *shalom* (meaning "peace"), or another sound or phrase that has special meaning to you.
- Continue for about 20 minutes.
- Bring yourself slowly back to normal consciousness. Do not jump up quickly. Become aware of your surroundings; stretch gently. Stand up and move around, slowly at first.

Counting meditation: Sitting comfortably, slowly count from one to ten in your head, keeping your attention on each number. If you feel your attention wandering (as undoubtedly it will), simply go back to one and start again.

Candle meditation: Sit in front of a lighted candle. Focus your eyes on the flame and keep your attention there.

Visualization/imagery: A relaxation technique related to meditation, visualization, or guided imagery, can help focus your mind on positive images to overcome negative emotions and manage stress. Sit or lie in a relaxed position and focus on your breathing, as for the basic meditation exercise. Then conjure up a peaceful and happy scene in your mind, visualizing yourself as part of it. Maintain a steady breathing rhythm and use your imagination to fill in as many details as you can of this tranquil scene.

Special precautions

Meditation occasionally produces negative effects. For example, the act of stilling the mind can sometimes bring up old, repressed memories. If you are already seeing a therapist, you may want to consult him or her before beginning meditation. If you have any frightening or disturbing experiences as a result of meditation, consult a trained counsellor or psychotherapist.

Position for meditation
The lotus and half-lotus yoga poses are popular for meditation because they provide a well-balanced, steady posture, but you should choose the position that is most comfortable for you.

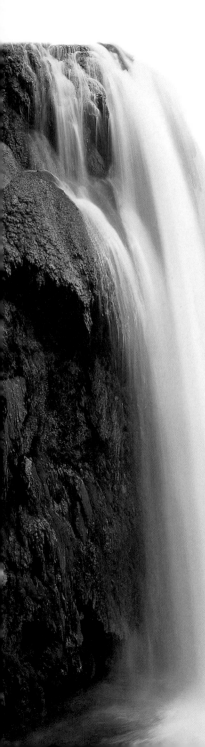

Naturopathy

This system of natural medicine emphasizes the value of restoring and promoting the human body's own self-healing processes. Naturopaths use a wide range of natural treatments, the most important of which are dietary management, herbal remedies, and a variety of physical therapies, such as hydrotherapy, which are selected according to the individual needs of the patient.

Beginning with the earliest civilizations, healers have made careful observations of the body in sickness and in health and used natural resources—food, water, air, and herbs—to help in the healing process. In the 19th century, a group of doctors began to develop this way of treating people into the science of naturopathy. The movement began in Europe and involved fasts, dietary regimes, baths, sprays, and compresses. As word of their success spread, these techniques were refined; in the early 20th century, they were introduced to America.

Life force
Most naturopathic doctors place emphasis on the therapeutic power of water, in the form of hot or cold baths, compresses, and spray treatments.

The naturopathic pioneers made many recommendations—such as the medicinal use of herbs and the consumption of more fresh vegetables, fruit, and wholegrain cereals—that have been borne out by modern research. The diets they designed are intended to rest the body from unhealthy foods, which increase the burden on the digestive processes and the body's detoxification and elimination systems, and to substitute foods that are easily processed and that strengthen the immune system. Today's naturopaths also often use water treatments and physical therapies to help the skin, lungs, intestines, and kidneys eliminate waste products that might otherwise hamper the healthy functioning of the body. Cold-water therapies are considered especially beneficial for boosting the effectiveness of the immune system.

The healing crisis

When you adopt a healthier lifestyle, eating more fresh natural foods, getting more exercise, and learning methods of relaxation, you may experience an improvement in general well-being. But after a few days or weeks, you may find that some of your old problems, such as colds or fatigue, return. Dr. Henry Lindlahr, the pioneering American naturopathic doctor, called this worsening of symptoms the healing crisis. He viewed it as a sign of the body increasing its normal ability to deal with toxins, infections, and waste products as it gains vitality. The symptoms usually clear in a few days with the help of appropriate naturopathic treatments.

Special precautions

If you are elderly, frail, or chronically sick, you may need to build up your vitality before being able to cope with the acute symptoms of a healing crisis (see facing page). In this case, consult a naturopath before trying any treatments on your own. Do not undertake naturopathic treatments without first seeking medical advice if you have epilepsy, diabetes, anaemia, unexplained weight loss, a psychiatric illness, or are pregnant or caring for a young child.

Consulting a professional

The naturopath gives you a thorough examination and asks you questions about your health, diet, lifestyle, likes, and dislikes. The purpose is to find out about your level of vitality and general health, as much as to diagnose any disease.

The practitioner may use laboratory tests, such as measuring mineral levels in your sweat or hair, essential fatty acids in your blood, or stress hormones in your saliva. He or she may also test the working of organs, such as your liver or pancreas, and check the permeability (leakiness) of the intestines. This will help build up a picture of the underlying causes of such problems as allergies, digestive disorders, headaches, chronic fatigue, hormone imbalances, and skin diseases. The naturopath may then recommend dietary changes, nutritional supplements, herbal treatments, or preparations that supplement digestive enzymes, such as pancreatin. Some practitioners are also trained in homeopathy (see pp. 38–41) and may prescribe remedies of this type. Many naturopaths are also qualified in some form of bodywork, such as osteopathy, and may use special soft-tissue massage techniques and gentle mobilization of joints—for example, to ease arthritic pain or improve breathing in people with asthma.

The practitioner may also prescribe some hydrotherapy treatments. Hydrotherapy involves a wide range of techniques that utilize water, from cold compresses to sitz baths (see below), showers, and sprays. These treatments are used to

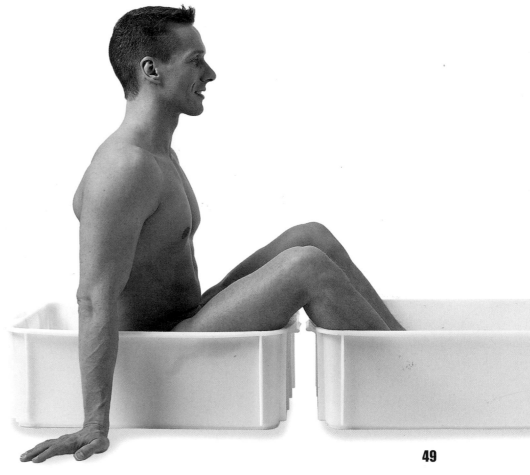

help relieve many disorders, from painful joints and menstrual problems to sore throats and feverish illnesses.

Using the therapy at home

Common ailments in people of any age respond very well to naturopathic medicine, and many of its treatments are easy to carry out at home. A major advantage of naturopathy is that its range of dietary and other remedies enables you to take more responsibility for your own health.

Naturopaths regard most acute symptoms—such as fevers, rashes, and diarrhoea—as positive signs of the body's defences at work (see box, p. 48). These symptoms generally need not be suppressed, but if you wish, you can help your body heal itself more quickly. Check the relevant pages in Part Two for specific advice on ailments.

Cold compress: Used to treat a wide variety of disorders, from joint strains and pains to headaches and bronchitis, cold compresses are generally applied to the affected area. Alternate hot and cold compresses are recommended for certain conditions (see Part Two). You will need a cotton handkerchief or piece of cloth for the compress itself; a towel, scarf, or bandage for the outer layer; and safety pins or bandage clips to keep the compress in place.

■ Select a piece of compress fabric of appropriate size—for throat, knee, wrist, or ankle, use a handkerchief; for the abdomen or trunk, use a sheet.
■ Soak the cloth in cold water, then wring it out and shake well.
■ Fold the material lengthwise and apply to the appropriate area.
■ Wrap the towel or other outer layer around the material and secure it in place with the safety pins or clips.
■ Keep the compress on for up to three hours or overnight. It should warm up within about 10

Body wrap

Use this treatment for colds and fevers. This type of compress should start to warm up within about 10 minutes. Test by putting your hand between the compress and the skin. If the compress is still cold, remove it and rub yourself vigorously with a dry towel.

1 Lay a towel on your bed or a mat on the floor. Place a folded sheet that has been wrung out in cold water over the towel, and lie on it.

2 Wrap the sheet around your abdomen, followed by the towel, and then pin together at the side.

minutes; if it remains cold, it may have been too wet, or your body may be too weak to respond satisfactorily, in which case the compress should be removed.

■ When you take off the compress, sponge the area with cool or lukewarm water to remove any perspiration.

■ You can use a similar technique to make a large compress to cover your waist or trunk (see facing page).

Hot or lukewarm baths: For this type of treatment, you can add healing ingredients to your bathwater, such as:

■ Two heaped tablespoons of Epsom salts (do not use if you have high blood pressure).

■ One heaped tablespoon of bicarbonate of soda.

■ Hayflowers (a bag of mixed, dried herbs, available from stores that stock herbs).

■ Aromatherapy oils (see pp. 28–31).

Cleansing diets: These short-term diets can help your body rid itself of waste products and environmental toxins. They eschew highly processed foods, which place a burden on the digestive system, and instead focus on raw foods. Naturopaths use cleansing diets (see box) for acute illnesses—such as colds, flu, bronchitis, gastroenteritis (for which soups and steamed vegetables may need to be used in place of raw salads)—and inflammatory disorders, such as skin rashes. Individual variations may need to be determined by a naturopath. Ideally you should consult a professional practitioner before beginning a cleansing diet. Some diets are unsuitable for children, the elderly, or those in poor health.

Three-day cleansing diet

Healthy people of most ages can follow this simple regimen for a limited period, but check with a health professional first.

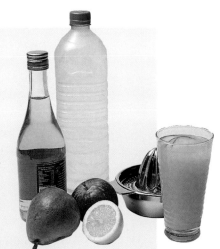

First day
Consume only pure fruit or vegetable juice. Use freshly extracted juices or canned or bottled unsweetened juices of apple, pear, grape, or pineapple (dilute 50 percent with water). Drink one glass four or five times daily. At other times drink pure spring water or boiled water with a teaspoon of lemon juice or apple-cider vinegar.

Second day
On rising and retiring or between meals, drink fruit juice or herbal tea (for example, lime tree flower, peppermint, chamomile). At meals eat fresh raw fruit (for example, grapes, apples, pears, peaches, melon, oranges). You can grate or cube hard fruit, and all may be mixed to make a fruit salad. Drink as much water as you like.

Third day
For breakfast have fresh or puréed fruit with live yogurt made from goat's or sheep's milk.

For lunch make a raw salad with a selection of leafy and grated root vegetables. Garnish with raisins and sunflower seeds. Eat fresh fruit for dessert.

For dinner eat vegetable soup or steamed vegetables flavoured with miso or soy sauce. Drink water when thirsty.

Reflexology

This natural therapy is based on the theory that there are certain "reflex points" on the hands and feet which correspond to the organs and other parts of the body. Applying pressure to these reflex points is said to produce many healing benefits, including stimulating the flow of energy through the body, improving nerve function and blood supply, releasing tension, and encouraging the organs of the body to work properly.

Reflexology has been practised for millennia in Western Asia, Japan, and China. In Egypt, drawings in the tomb of Ankamahor at Saqqara—known as the Physician's Tomb—show the therapy being performed on the feet and hands. These pictures date back to 2330 B.C.

In the West, reflexology dates from the early 20th century. American doctor William Fitzgerald described 10 channels of communication, running vertically through the body from the feet and hands to the brain. Fitzgerald found that he could anaesthetize the face, head, and neck by means of pressure applied to the fingers. Fitzgerald's follower Eunice Ingham developed his work, performing reflexology on thousands of pairs of feet and finding out which parts of the feet correspond to which organs of the body.

Today foot reflexology is one of the most popular forms of complementary medicine, though its healing powers are not scientifically proven. Many people report it to be of benefit in a host of common everyday ailments—from sinusitis to irritable bowel syndrome, menstrual problems to back pain—and believe that it has powerful effects in relieving tension in the body.

Consulting a professional

The reflexologist will work on each foot, paying special attention to areas that are tender or painful (this is believed to indicate a blockage of

Giving treatment

The person receiving treatment should be seated on a comfortable chair with the leg of the foot being treated supported on a stool or a large pillow. To administer the therapy, either kneel on the floor or sit on a low chair or stool. Work across the sole, front, and sides of the feet using your thumb or index finger. Because you are contacting tiny reflex points, move your thumb or finger forwards slowly, using controlled, deep pressure. The forward movement should be like the creeping motion of a caterpillar.

The thumb technique
Use your thumb for the soles and sides of the feet. Wrap one hand around the toes and apply controlled, deep pressure using the inside edge of the thumb of the other hand. Bend the thumb joint slightly and "walk" the thumb forwards by bending and straightening the joint.

The index finger technique
Use your index finger for the tops and sides of the feet. Press with the index finger, again "walking" it forwards by alternately bending and unbending the first joint. Use your thumb and other three fingers for support.

Special precautions

Reflexology is generally safe for all age groups, but do not use it if the feet have open sores or signs of infection, inflammation, or athlete's foot. Also avoid reflexology if you have diabetes or varicose veins or if you are or might be pregnant.

energy in the corresponding part of the body). He or she will apply pressure to the relevant reflex points to free congestion and aid healing.

Using this therapy at home

Before trying reflexology, be sure to seek medical advice if the cause of symptoms is unknown. You can treat yourself, but practitioners believe that having someone else work on your reflex points greatly expands the range of benefits. If problems continue after treatment, consult your doctor.

The right position
The person giving reflexology supports the heel in his free hand while working on the underside of the foot.

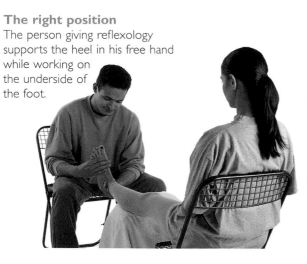

Reflexology foot maps

The reflexes on the left and right soles are similar, with points for many parts of the body appearing on both feet (indicated with an asterisk in the illustration below). But some organs have points on one sole only, usually reflecting the side of the body on which the organ is situated.

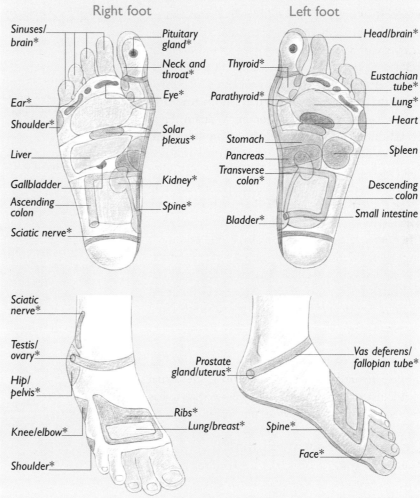

Right foot

Sinuses/brain*
Pituitary gland*
Neck and throat*
Eye*
Ear*
Shoulder*
Solar plexus*
Liver
Gallbladder
Kidney*
Ascending colon
Spine*
Sciatic nerve*

Left foot

Head/brain*
Thyroid*
Eustachian tube*
Parathyroid*
Lung*
Heart
Stomach
Pancreas
Spleen
Transverse colon*
Descending colon
Bladder*
Small intestine

Sciatic nerve*
Testis/ovary*
Hip/pelvis*
Prostate gland/uterus*
Vas deferens/fallopian tube*
Ribs*
Lung/breast*
Spine*
Knee/elbow*
Face*
Shoulder*

Yoga

The ancient Indian tradition of yoga involves a wide variety of mind–body exercises, which range from postural and breathing exercises to deep relaxation and meditation. Yoga therapy tailors these exercises to the requirements of individuals with health problems. Besides helping to treat particular disorders, regular yoga practice also boosts energy levels and improves all-round health and well-being.

Yoga therapy springs from the rich, age-old tradition of yoga, which emerged on the Indian subcontinent thousands of years ago. The philosophy behind yoga encompasses every level of existence, from the physical to the spiritual. However, if you prefer, it is possible to disconnect yoga from spiritual teaching and work on improving your physical and mental health.

Indian doctors have long relied on yoga. But today's yoga therapy, pioneered by Swami Kuvalayananda in Bombay during the early 1920s, is a relatively new discipline, marrying traditional yoga and modern medicine. In the decades following its inception, the therapy spread to other parts of India. Today, many of the country's yoga therapy clinics are associated with hospitals.

In the West, psychologists and doctors now widely use relaxation techniques derived from yoga for the treatment of anxiety and stress. They

Ultimate relaxation
The Sanskrit name for the yoga position shown below is *savasana*, which means "corpse pose". It provides physical stillness, encouraging mental calm. Lie on your back with blankets under your head and back. Draw your feet apart, allowing them to roll outwards. Rest your arms, hands palms-up, away from your sides. Close your eyes and relax.

Breathing awareness

Breathing is one of the few bodily processes that are governed by both the central and autonomic nervous systems. In other words, it is controlled automatically, so that you can continuously breathe without thinking about it, but you can also intervene consciously in your breathing patterns. This provides a very important link between mind and body. Yoga uses exercises to correct poor breathing patterns, which can have profound effects on general health and on particular disorders, such as asthma and anxiety. Try the following basic breathing exercise:

1 Lie down in the corpse pose (see photograph), with folded blankets placed under your head and back.

2 Close your eyes, but keep your gaze turned downwards towards your chest. Relax and notice how your breathing slows.

3 Be aware of your breath entering and leaving your body. Notice the changing temperature of the air and feel how it passes into your body.

4 Listen to the soft sounds of your breathing and, at the same time, pay particular attention to the differences between your inhalation and your exhalation.

are also beginning to recognize the value of yoga's postural, breathing, relaxation, and meditation exercises for the treatment of many other common conditions, such as arthritis, heart disease, high blood pressure, migraine, obesity, and premenstrual syndrome.

Consulting a professional

A yoga therapist assesses your health problems together with your constitution, lifestyle, stress level, and other general health factors. He or she then selects yoga techniques that are most suited to your condition and teaches them to you either individually or in a small, specialized class. At the same time, the therapist devises a yoga session for your daily practice at home. He or she will revise this regimen as your skills develop and your condition responds.

Because yoga therapy seeks to establish harmony between mind, body, and spirit, your regimen should include a balanced set of practices that calm and vitalize you both mentally and physically, as well as working on specific ailments. The yoga techniques used in therapy work are often surprisingly simple, and a skilled therapist will be able to devise a programme that you can start to put into practice without difficulty, whatever your condition.

Using the therapy at home

Yoga's effectiveness depends on frequent, regular practice, even if only for a short period each day. You should therefore develop a yoga routine that suits your lifestyle as well as your particular health problems. This session should not be too long, so that you can easily integrate it into your daily life.

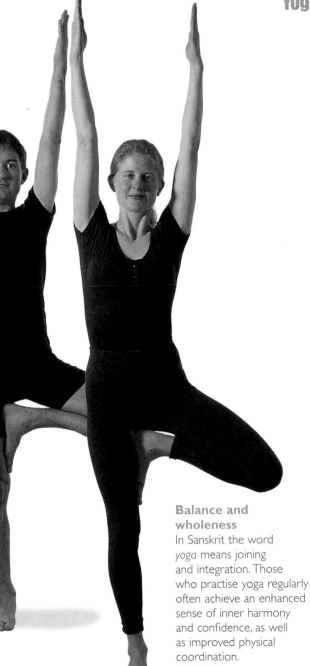

Balance and wholeness
In Sanskrit the word *yoga* means joining and integration. Those who practise yoga regularly often achieve an enhanced sense of inner harmony and confidence, as well as improved physical coordination.

The best way to create your yoga programme is to consult a qualified yoga therapist, or a yoga teacher if no therapist is available locally. Books and videos can help you to learn yoga, but they are no substitute for a good teacher. There are many subtle aspects of yoga practice that cannot be adequately learned without an expert to observe and advise you. Particular postures to address specific health needs are even more helpful when integrated into a structured session of yoga exercises, which may include a variety of postures, breathing exercises, and relaxation and meditation techniques.

Practice tips

- Find a quiet place in an uncluttered, well-ventilated room.
- Wear non-restrictive clothing, and place a non-slip mat or a blanket on the floor to make yourself more comfortable.
- Use folded blankets as padding for your head and back when doing postures that require lying down.
- Avoid bright lights, distractions, and interruptions.
- Establish a regular time for your yoga session before

Serene moments
One of the goals of yoga is to allow life energy, or *prana*, to flow freely through body and mind.

breakfast, lunch, or dinner. If this is not possible, do your yoga practice at least one hour after a snack or three and a half hours after a main meal.

Although mild ailments such as aching shoulders may be resolved by just a few minutes of daily practice, more entrenched conditions, such as asthma, usually require longer sessions. You may have to continue these for many months. However, even short-term practice will often yield significant improvements.

Postures: Yoga positions (or *asanas*) work to relax, strengthen, and vitalize every part of your body. They often target the spine, bending it forwards, backwards, and sideways, and rotating it in both directions. They work the body's joints through their full range of motion, thus helping to maintain flexibility. And they improve breathing by releasing tension in the muscles of the rib cage. Because of the close interrelation between body and mind, these actions on the body will also affect the mind, thereby helping to reduce the effects of stress and emotional discord.

Relaxation: Deep relaxation can dispel states of stress and fatigue within minutes. It can also benefit a wide range of disorders, such as migraine and irritable bowel syndrome, that may be triggered by the release of chemicals in the body in response to anxiety. Yoga relaxation is usually carried out lying motionless on your back (see p. 54). A variety of techniques are used. In most cases these involve focusing your awareness on parts of the body, on your breathing, or on mental images.

Meditation, a technique related to yoga, involves slowing down your thoughts and enhancing awareness (see p. 46).

Special precautions

You should always practise yoga in a gentle manner. It should not cause pain or discomfort. When practised in this way, yoga is very safe. However, there are a number of ailments for which particular yoga postures may be unsuitable or even dangerous. When in doubt, consult your doctor. Examples of these conditions are listed below.

- **Abdominal hernia:** Avoid postures (for example, prone postures) that increase pressure in the abdomen.
- **Arthritis:** Avoid exercising inflamed joints.
- **Back or neck pain:** Avoid any posture that increases the pain, either during the yoga session or afterwards.
- **Chronic bronchitis and emphysema:** Avoid strenuous exercises.
- **Depression:** Deep relaxation and meditation can help in some cases but may exacerbate the condition in others.
- **Epilepsy:** Avoid breathing techniques that may increase the aeration of the lungs, for example, rapid abdominal breathing or deep breathing, unless practised under expert supervision.
- **High blood pressure (hypertension):** Avoid inverted postures, strenuous exercises, and any exercise involving breath-holding.
- **Heart disease:** Seek advice from a qualified yoga therapist.
- **Obesity:** Avoid inverted postures and the plough.

Using a mat
A yoga mat provides a safe, non-slip surface on which to practise. Ask your teacher for advice on where to buy one.

Glossary of Therapies

This glossary lists the most popular natural therapies that cannot generally be undertaken without the help of an expert therapist. (For advice on finding a suitable therapist, see p. 17.) They vary widely in their acceptance by orthodox doctors, so each therapy is given a star rating as a rough guide to how it is valued by the medical profession.

> **MEDICAL RATING KEY**
> Very high ★★★★ Average ★★
> High ★★★ Low ★

ACUPUNCTURE ★★★
Part of the system of traditional Chinese medicine, acupuncture aims to restore the body to a state of health and balance by regulating the flow of energy (known as *qi*, pronounced "chee") along a series of lines, called meridians, that are believed to run through the body. Acupuncturists do this mainly by inserting fine needles into the skin at certain points on the meridians. Each point is thought to affect a particular organ or function. Acupuncturists claim to be able to treat a wide variety of diseases, including anxiety and depression, musculoskeletal problems, high blood pressure and circulation problems, menstrual and menopausal symptoms, headaches, allergic rhinitis, and back pain.

Professional consultation
On your first visit, the therapist takes a detailed medical history and asks you questions about your lifestyle. He or she examines your tongue and skin tone and takes your 12 meridian pulses—6 on each wrist. Most people need further visits, the number depending on the particular problem.

The most common form of treatment is insertion of needles. This is usually painless, although you may feel a slight tingle. The needles are left in place for a time ranging from a few minutes to a half hour. You may also be given other treatments, such as acupressure (see pp. 24–27) and moxibustion (the burning of a herb called moxa over an acupuncture point).

ALEXANDER TECHNIQUE ★★★★
The aim of the Alexander technique is to improve your posture and the way you move and carry out everyday actions in order to reduce effort and muscle tension and improve overall health. The technique was devised by an Australian actor, Frederick Matthias Alexander (1869–1955).

Professional consultation
When you begin a series of Alexander lessons, the teacher assesses the way you stand, sit, and move. He or she then uses gentle manipulation to show you what the best posture and body movements feel like. You are also told how to encourage good posture and movement and how to discourage tension between lessons.

Many Alexander students feel better after their first lesson, but most need about 25 lessons before they achieve lasting results. Teachers have reported benefits to people who suffer from a range of disorders, including digestive problems, heart and circulation disorders, breathing difficulties, gynaecological conditions, and back pain.

ANTHROPOSOPHICAL MEDICINE ★
This form of medicine relies on the theory that each person has four systems that must be kept in balance: the physical body, the astral body (said to control the senses and emotional life), the etheric body (responsible for growth), and the ego (a person's consciousness of self).

Anthroposophical doctors are qualified in orthodox medicine but prefer to draw on a range of treatments, including herbal and homeopathic medicines, massage, and creative therapies, whenever possible. With this broad approach, anthroposophical medicine claims to be able to deal with all types of ailments.

AUTOGENIC TRAINING ★★★
This system provides a highly effective way of relaxing and of surviving stress. It can help prevent stress-related illnesses of many kinds, as well as being beneficial in treating different types of addiction.

A qualified practitioner leads you through exercises designed to induce different physiological states that bring about relaxation. These states include feelings of warmth, the sensation of heaviness, concentration on the heartbeat, calm breathing, and the sensation of cold on the forehead.

Auricular therapy

In this branch of acupuncture, needles are inserted into points on the ear. Auricular therapists see the ear as a mirror of the whole body, with acupuncture points relating to each organ and function. Some therapists also use small electrical charges, or magnetic ball bearings to stimulate the points.

AYURVEDIC MEDICINE ★★

The traditional Indian form of healing is called Ayurvedic medicine. Its basic premise is that health depends on a balance between the five basic elements, known as the *doshas*, each of which governs five body systems: ether (networks and channels within the body), earth (solid parts, such as bones), water (soft tissue and fluids), fire (the digestive system), and air (the nervous system and senses). The energy (*prana*) that connects them is also very important.

Professional consultation

The therapist aims to find out about as many as possible of the factors that can affect your health, from your lifestyle and medical history to your astrological chart. Once the practitioner has examined you, taken your pulse, and asked you about your health, he or she may prescribe such treatments as detoxification (using steam, baths, and essential oils), massage, and herbal medicines. You will also be given advice about your diet, and the therapist may recommend yoga or some other suitable form of exercise. Ayurvedic doctors look on the therapy as a system of medicine that can be used for any complaint. You may need a number of return visits, especially if you have a long-standing illness or health problem.

BATES METHOD ★

This system of exercises, devised by Dr. William H. Bates (1860–1931), is designed to improve poor eyesight. The exercises are based on the idea that eyesight problems are often the result of the poor functioning of muscles around the eyes. Eye disorders such as far- and nearsightedness, squinting, and astigmatism may respond to regular practice of Bates method exercises.

BIOCHEMIC TISSUE SALTS ★

Therapy with biochemic tissue salts is based on treatment with pills containing minerals in highly dilute form. The minute amounts of minerals contained in these pills makes many orthodox doctors sceptical of the effectiveness of this form of therapy.

BIOENERGETICS ★

This therapy relies on the idea that a "life force" flows through the body and mind. If the flow is interrupted, illness can result. Therapists aim to unblock the flow of life energy, relieving tension and bringing emotional release. Practitioners claim success with anxiety and depression and with those affected by Down's syndrome and autism.

Professional consultation

Bioenergetics begins with a one-to-one consultation with your practitioner. He or she assesses your problem and recommends a series of exercises designed to unblock your energy. Later, you may join a group session in which you can practise the exercises.

BIOFEEDBACK ★★★★

This technique provides a way of measuring changes in the body, such as skin temperature and muscle tension. It is possible to use the power of thought to alter some of these changes, and this becomes easier when you can see the results on a meter or screen. Since many physical changes are related to illness, it is sometimes possible to treat the disease as well. For example, some people have been able to ease the pain of migraine by

---

Biodynamics

Biodynamics works in a similar way to bioenergetics but is based on the idea that the digestive system reacts to your moods and emotions. Therapists use massage to treat the digestive system, and look on a rumbling stomach as a sign that treatment is working.

---

imagining the head getting cooler. Biofeedback can also be effective against stress-related problems like asthma, high blood pressure, insomnia, and anxiety.

Professional consultation

After instructing you in a specific relaxation technique, such as focusing on your health, the therapist shows you how to read the meters and how to recognize changes in your nervous system. The goal is to help you bring on a state of relaxation yourself.

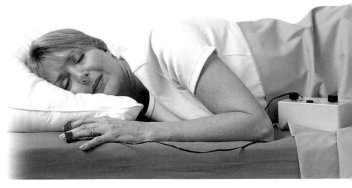

The Therapies

BIORHYTHMS ★
The theory behind biorhythms is that there are three fixed-length cycles that affect your health and performance in different areas of life. The physical cycle lasts 23 days and governs such areas as vitality, the immune system, confidence, and sex drive. The emotional cycle lasts 28 days and affects creativity and moods. The intellectual cycle lasts 33 days and influences mental function.

Advocates of this theory believe it is possible to plot the biorhythms for your entire life, starting with your birth, as a series of graphs. Special computer programs are available to do this. When a particular cycle is at its peak, your performance and energy in that area are said to be at their highest; troughs indicate passive periods. You can use biorhythms to plan events in your life, scheduling important events that require high performance on days when one or more of your rhythms is high.

BUTEYKO BREATHING ★★
This therapy is based on the work of Konstantin Buteyko, a Russian scientist. Its premise is that breathing too rapidly can cause chemical changes in the blood that result in various health problems, including anxiety, muscle tension, headaches, dizziness, and asthma. When you attend a Buteyko breathing course, you perform exercises in breathing slowly and holding your breath. Some asthma sufferers have been able to reduce their need for drug treatment after learning Buteyko breathing, but the therapy should be undertaken only in consultation with your doctor. People with asthma should not adjust their medication except on the advice of a medical practitioner.

CHI KUNG (QI GONG) ★★★
The term chi kung means "internal energy exercise". An ancient Chinese system of exercises, chi kung aims to stimulate the flow of energy, which Chinese physicians believe travels around the body along channels known as meridians. The therapy concentrates on your posture and breathing and teaches you how to focus your mind. There are also chi kung healers who try to use the energy to cure illnesses.

Many different forms of chi kung exist, but, in contrast to some Western exercise regimes, they are all gentle. Tai chi chuan (see p. 65) is one well-known form of chi kung.

CHINESE MEDICINE ★★
Traditional Chinese doctors use herbs along with techniques such as acupuncture, diet, and exercise to provide a complete system of medical treatment. The goal is to regulate the flow through the body of the vital energy called *qi*. The therapist examines you as a whole person (taking into account the health of your mind, body, and spirit)— examining your hair, eyes, skin, and tongue, as well as taking your pulse.

The practitioner will recommend a treatment programme to suit your particular symptoms rather than to cure a specific ailment.

> ## Zhan zhuang
> A powerful and popular form of chi kung is called zhan zhuang (which means "standing like a tree"). To do zhan zhuang exercises, you adopt a series of different stationary positions, which may involve lying down, sitting, or standing.

Chinese physicians prescribe from a wide variety of herbs, including some, such as ginseng and ginkgo, that are now well-known in the West. They are selected for properties such as their ability to warm, cool, affect specific organs of the body, and regulate the flow of *qi*. For example, cooling herbs might be prescribed if you have a high temperature. You will usually be asked to make several return visits so that the therapist can review the treatment. As Chinese herbalism is part of a complete medical system, practitioners claim to be able to treat a wide range of disorders.

CHIROPRACTIC ★★★
Chiropractic is a manipulative therapy, primarily designed to treat disorders of the muscles and bones, especially the joints. The therapy began as a way of treating diseases by manipulating the bones of the spine, but modern chiropractors treat a wide range of musculo-skeletal problems. People with joint problems, especially back pain, often report good results

from chiropractic treatment. Other conditions—such as arthritis, rheumatism, migraine, and asthma—have also responded well to this form of therapy.

Professional consultation

When you first visit a chiropractor, he or she examines you thoroughly, feels your spine, and tests the mobility of your joints. The practitioner may also take X rays of your spine and check your blood pressure. He or she may then use gentle manipulative techniques on your joints and may also massage your muscles. The chiropractor may give you advice about exercises to help the mobility of your joints.

CLINICAL ECOLOGY ★★

Also known as environmental medicine, clinical ecology attempts to heal illnesses that result from our surroundings. Clinical ecologists treat people who suffer from allergies to foods and those who are adversely affected by chemicals in the environment, such as pesticides and petrol fumes.

A range of disorders may be caused by allergies and similar reactions. Clinical ecologists claim to be able to help people with asthma, headaches, psoriasis and eczema, repeated stomach upsets, long-standing fatigue, and rheumatoid arthritis.

Professional consultation

The therapist may test blood, urine, and, occasionally, hair—to detect your responses to different substances. For food sensitivities the simplest method of diagnosis is an exclusion diet, in which you eat only a small number of different foods, gradually adding others until you find one that causes an

adverse reaction (see also "Food Sensitivity", pp. 212–215). Using the information gathered from the various methods of analysis, the clinical ecologist will recommend a diet or lifestyle that helps you avoid foods or substances that make you ill.

COLOUR THERAPY ★

This therapy involves treatment with particular colours of light, applied in a variety of ways. It is based on the idea that certain wavelengths of light have healing effects on specific parts of the body or on the mind. Therapists claim to be able to treat many disorders, including depression, stress, learning difficulties, and skin problems.

The therapist takes your medical history and asks you about your colour preferences. He or she then suggests treatment. This may involve basking in coloured lights, wearing clothes of certain colours, eating foods of a particular colour, or drinking water that has been treated with coloured light.

CRANIAL OSTEOPATHY ★★

This branch of osteopathy involves gentle manipulation of the bones of the skull (cranium). A cranial osteopath may also work on your shoulders and spine to help the joints and tissues to move freely. Cranial osteopaths believe that if these bones or the nearby tissues are shifted even slightly out of place— for example, by an injury—health problems may develop throughout the body. Cranial osteopaths therefore claim to be able to provide benefit not only for head and spinal injuries, mouth and jaw pain, and sinusitis, but also for ailments affecting other parts of the body, such as arthritis, constipation, menstrual problems, and migraine.

CREATIVE THERAPIES ★★★

The use of the arts—such as painting, drawing, music, and dance—can have powerful healing effects. Emotions that are too deep for words can come to the surface through creative expression, helping people overcome difficult feelings, aiding relaxation, and ideally leading to greater physical well-being. Creative therapies have been found especially effective for people with emotional problems, particularly those who find it difficult to communicate their feelings to others. Dance therapy has the additional benefit of providing physical exercise.

CRYSTAL THERAPY ★

Practitioners of this therapy believe that crystals and gemstones produce different types of healing energy. Crystal therapists arrange crystals around you or place them on your body, choosing stones that are thought to be effective for your problem.

FELDENKRAIS METHOD ★★

This is a technique—influenced by yoga, martial arts, and the Alexander technique— that aims to help you move with ease, using minimal effort and maximum efficiency. Teachers of the Feldenkrais method try to make you more aware of your body movements, recognizing any tensions and correcting them by changing the way you move. They do this by teaching you simple exercises to change your habitual patterns of movement, and by using touch to direct you towards less stressful, and therefore less damaging, ways of moving your body. Teachers of the method claim that it can help people suffering from back pain, paralysis, and the after-effects of a stroke.

The Therapies

FENG SHUI ★

The ancient Chinese art of placement, or feng shui, relies on the theory that, like the human body, the earth is crisscrossed by a series of channels, along which flows vital energy, or *qi*. Practitioners of feng shui believe that the design and position of a building and the way its contents are chosen and arranged can affect the flow of *qi*, and thus make the building a more auspicious and healthier place in which to live. If you consult a feng shui practitioner, he or she will take readings with a special compass and assess the rooms of your home using Chinese astrology and the ancient *I Ching* ("Book of Changes"). The practitioner may then recommend alterations, such as moving mirrors and other items and rearranging the furnishings. Exponents claim such changes may improve psychological and physical well-being.

FLOTATION THERAPY ★★

A method of relaxation, flotation therapy involves floating in a large tank filled with water containing a high concentration of Epsom salts. You wear earplugs, the lights are switched off, and the water is kept at the same temperature as your skin. The result is that all outside sensations are removed, and most people, even many who are highly stressed, relax deeply within minutes.

Flotation therapy may help stress-related problems, such as anxiety, migraines, and headaches. People with back pain and muscle fatigue may also benefit. The therapy tends to reduce pain because it stimulates the body to release its own natural painkillers, hormone-like substances called endorphins. Some people even experience euphoria.

HEALING ★★

Healers usually talk about what they do in terms of energy—a vital life force, which everyone possesses. This force can become depleted when someone is ill, but healers believe that they can transfer vital energy to a sick person. There are many different types of healing, including faith healing, which is based on a religious faith shared by healer and patient, and spiritual healing, in which the healing energy is separate from the beliefs of the people taking part. Reiki (p. 65) is a form of healing therapy.

Some studies indicate that healing can be beneficial. It may help to relieve pain, or, by providing comfort, it may help the person to cope with the illness more effectively, even though the actual disease remains.

Professional consultation
Healers work in a variety of ways. Some attempt to transfer their "healing energy" through their hands, touching you gently. Some hold their hands an inch or so away from your skin. Others channel healing energy by thinking or praying. You may feel

> ## Therapeutic touch
>
> Practitioners of therapeutic touch believe that every human being has an energy force that extends outside the body. When this force is blocked or out of balance, illness results. Practitioners try to correct these problems by passing their hands over the sick person (sometimes without touching). One session of such healing takes 10–15 minutes.

a sensation of warmth as the practitioner places his or her hands on or near your body. A reputable healer may advise you to consult your doctor as well as undergoing healing. Beware of any healer who makes promises to cure or prevent disease, who charges an exorbitant fee, or who challenges your religious faith.

HELLERWORK ★

Practitioners of Hellerwork believe that the bones and soft tissues of the body become misaligned from stress, illness, or bad posture. Hellerworkers aim to realign your body, banish tension, and correct the problems that originally caused the misalignment. They do this by manipulating the body and by teaching you how to move in a well-balanced way. People with a wide range of aches and pains, especially neck ache, back pain, and headaches, have responded well to this form of therapy. It may also help internal processes affected by muscle function, such as digestive problems.

Professional consultation
You normally attend a series of 11 weekly sessions, making up a complete Hellerwork course. After taking your medical history and assessing your needs, the practitioner will begin the first group of sessions, known as the superficial sessions. These concentrate on freeing tension in the chest, arms, and feet. Next come the core sessions, during which the therapist works on muscles that Hellerworkers believe to be at the core of the body—those of the pelvis, spine, head, and neck. A final group of sessions, known as the integrative sessions, draws together the work of the previous weeks.

HYPNOTHERAPY ★★

This therapy uses hypnosis, creating a state of mind in which normal thought processes are suspended for a short period of time. Hypnosis can be used to induce relaxation, to treat stress-related conditions, to help people overcome addictions, phobias, and eating disorders, and to treat a lack of confidence and sexual problems. Some forms of hypnosis are also effective for pain relief, especially during labour and dental treatment.

Professional consultation

There are various ways of inducing a hypnotic trance, but the hypnotist will create a relaxing atmosphere, perhaps asking you to visualize a restful scene or repeat a phrase or sentence over and over. The therapist may suggest that your limbs are feeling heavy and that your eyelids are closing. When you go into a hypnotic trance, you will feel relaxed and you may be willing to accept the suggestions of the hypnotist. You may then go into a deeper trance, in which your heartbeat and breathing slow down and you enter a state that feels similar to that of meditation (see pp. 46–47). The hypnotist may make statements to address your problem—for example, ones that boost your self-esteem or tell you that you are going to stop a damaging form of behaviour, such as smoking or drinking alcohol.

IRIDOLOGY ★

A technique said to help diagnose diseases, iridology is based on the idea that the iris of the eye contains a map of the body. Each part of the iris is believed to represent an organ. Iridologists believe that black marks on the irises indicate a disease and white marks signal some form of stress or inflammation. If an iridologist believes you have a problem, he or she will refer you to a doctor.

KINESIOLOGY ★

Like Chinese physicians, kinesiologists believe that an invisible form of vital energy circulates through the body. Treatment aims to restore imbalances in this energy flow. A kinesiologist tries to learn about your health by testing your muscles, and tries to correct imbalances of the muscles and other disorders by gentle massage, acupressure, and similar physical techniques.

Kinesiology can sometimes relieve muscular aches and pains. Practitioners also claim success in treating food sensitivities, although there is no evidence supporting these claims.

Professional consultation

The therapist will ask you about your medical history and health problems. He or she will then test your muscles by pressing them carefully, and will gently massage areas where the energy flow is thought to be blocked. The kinesiologist may touch acupressure points lightly or stimulate these points with an electrical device. He or she may also test your reactions to various foods and recommend dietary changes.

LAUGHTER THERAPY ★★

When you laugh, you feel good. The reason for this is partly that laughter boosts certain body chemicals, including endorphins, which are natural mood-enhancing and pain-relieving substances. There is also evidence that laughter has physical benefits—it relaxes tense muscles and strengthens the immune system. A number of therapists run workshops in which you are encouraged to laugh—for example, by watching a clown, listening to a comedian, or being shown the funny side of problems. This can make your difficulties seem more manageable, so laughter therapy can also provide a way of managing stress.

LIGHT THERAPY ★★★

One of the many forms of this therapy involves sitting in front of a specially designed light box, which produces light at a much higher intensity than ordinary bulbs. This helps many sufferers of winter seasonal affective disorder (SAD), or winter blues. These people suffer depression during the winter months because of high levels of the hormone melatonin, which is produced by the pineal gland. The gland normally produces melatonin at night; the morning light makes it stop secreting the hormone. But during winter, when there is less daylight, the pineal gland may go on producing melatonin. About two hours of light therapy on a daily basis may help to alleviate the problem.

MAGNET THERAPY ★

This therapy relies on the idea that the body responds to magnetism. The therapist applies magnets to your body, either in the form of a magnetic bracelet or as magnetic pads. Therapists claim success in treating the pain of rheumatism, but most research has shown that magnets have little or no therapeutic effect, and experts are therefore sceptical.

METAMORPHIC TECHNIQUE ★

This therapy involves work on the feet and hands, using techniques similar to reflexology (see pp. 52–53). Just as reflexologists believe that different zones on the feet affect different parts of the body, so practitioners of the metamorphic technique believe that various areas on the feet affect the emotions.

NUTRITIONAL THERAPY ★★★★

This form of therapy analyses your diet and finds ways in which your body's strength and ability to heal itself can be improved by making changes in your eating habits. Besides dietitians and nutritional therapists, practitioners such as clinical ecologists and naturopaths often use nutritional therapy as part of their treatment.

When you first consult a nutritional therapist, you fill in a questionnaire about your health, illnesses, lifestyle, and diet. After the therapist has looked at your answers, he or she gives you dietary advice tailored to your particular situation. You should expect to make return visits so that the therapist can assess the diet's effectiveness and make any necessary adjustments. The practitioner may also advise you to consult your doctor if you have a condition that cannot be treated solely by dietary means.

OSTEOPATHY ★★★★

This system of medicine treats the mechanics of the human body—the bones, joints, muscles, ligaments, and other connective tissues. Osteopaths believe that many diseases are due to problems with the body's structure; therefore, fixing the structural problems helps the body heal itself. They use gentle, manipulative techniques such as massage, manipulation and advice on posture to reduce tension and restore health. Although

osteopathy is especially effective in treating problems such as muscle and joint pains, an osteopath always tries to find out why these disorders occur, in case they are symptoms of some other disorder.

Professional consultation

A first visit usually lasts up to one hour. The osteopath asks about your lifestyle, work, and leisure activities, as well as your illness. He or she examines you standing, sitting, and lying on the treatment table. You may be asked to bend or stretch to see how your body responds in different positions.

Soft-tissue manipulation, with a range of massage-like techniques that help relax tight muscles and tighten loose ones, is often the first stage in treatment. The osteopath uses his or her fingertips to probe your muscles to seek out tension and other problems.

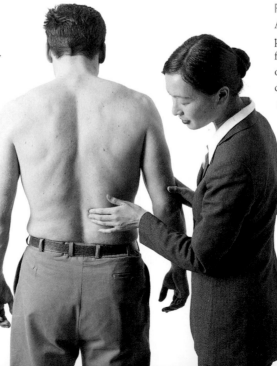

If you have joint problems, the osteopath may use gentle rhythmic strokes and stretches to ease them. He or she may also try a technique known as the high-velocity thrust. This is a rapid, painless movement, usually used on the spine. It makes the joint move and click and the muscles around the joint quickly relax. Pain around the joint can be relieved with this technique.

You may require several return visits, which usually last about half an hour each. The number needed will vary according to several factors—the condition itself, how long you have had the problem, and your age (younger people usually need fewer visits).

Besides joint and muscle problems, disorders that may respond well to osteopathy include sports injuries, migraine, premenstrual syndrome, constipation, and respiratory problems such as asthma.

POLARITY THERAPY ★

A mixture of Eastern and Western approaches, polarity therapy is based on the idea that a form of energy flows around the body from one pole to another, rather like a magnetic current. The energy, which may be positive, negative, or neutral, flows between energy centres known, as in yoga, as *chakras*. Polarity therapists use four techniques to balance energy and promote general health: bodywork (touch and massage), awareness skills (helping you talk through your problems), dietary recommendations, and stretching exercises (a series of yoga-like postures).

PSYCHOTHERAPY ★★★★

Trained to listen carefully and offer support in cases of distress, grief, stress, and anxiety, psychotherapists treat many people with emotional and psychological problems. Therapists work by listening to you and talking with you about your experiences and relationships, so that you can gain insight into your problems. Gradually, you get closer to the roots of emotional difficulties that may be deep-seated.

Psychotherapists use a variety of different therapies, ranging from the warm and supportive to the more detached and analytical. When choosing a therapist, it is important to find out which technique he or she offers. Some of the most popular are behavioural therapy (which helps you "unlearn" problem behaviour or habits), group therapy (in which you share your problems with a group of other patients), neurolinguistic programming (which works with the way personal experiences influence your perceptions), and gestalt therapy (which makes you more aware of behaviour such as body language).

Depending on the type of therapy and the needs of the patient, psychotherapy may be short-term or may require a large number of sessions over months or even years. After a course of therapy, you should be able to confront and overcome your difficulties.

REIKI ★

The word *reiki* means "universal life energy", and this therapy offers a way of transferring healing energy from a giver to a receiver. Practitioners gain their ability to heal through reiki by studying with a reiki master teacher. The student practitioner undergoes "attunement", which is said to open up a channel through which healing energy can flow. Practitioners also learn specific hand positions for use during therapy sessions.

When you consult a reiki practitioner, the therapist lays his or her hands on your body, following their intuition to adopt the positions that give the best flow of healing energy.

ROLFING ★

The aim of rolfing is to improve the structural alignment of the body. Rolfers compare the human body to a tower of children's building blocks—if one block is pushed out of alignment, the structure of the entire tower is threatened. By manipulating the body's connective tissues and muscles— using the knuckles, fingers, palms, and elbows—the rolfer tries to realign your body, increasing range of movement, improving balance, and enhancing posture. Rolfing may be of benefit to people with poor posture and low vitality.

SOUND THERAPY ★★

Scientists now know that sound can alter our brainwaves. This therapy uses the power of sound to encourage healing. Treatment may be a simple matter of playing soothing sounds (such as chanting, the noise of waves, or the calls of dolphins) to induce relaxation. This type of sound therapy can be effective when used to combat stress, anxiety, and other emotional problems.

TAI CHI CHUAN ★★★

Performed as a series of graceful postures, one flowing into another, the Chinese "soft" martial art of tai chi chuan—or simply tai chi—works on both the body, by providing exercise, and the mind, by helping you concentrate. The movements relax the muscles, freeing the joints and easing tension. Tai chi provides gentle exercise suitable for most people.

Professional consultation

The best way to learn tai chi is to go to a class run by an experienced teacher. You will learn a sequence of movements known as a "form"—either a short form, lasting 5 to 10 minutes, or a full-length long form, which can take up to 40 minutes. Once you have learned a tai chi form, you will be able to practise it every day at home.

TIBETAN MEDICINE ★

The native medicine of Tibet is based on the theory that the body contains three substances called humours—vital energy, internal heat, and phlegm. In a healthy person, these substances are balanced, but when they are imbalanced, they turn into three poisons— desire, anger, and greed—and illness results.

When you consult a practitioner of Tibetan medicine, he or she will manipulate the artery in the wrist so as to feel the pulse in three different ways, examine a urine sample, ask you about your lifestyle and habits, and draw up your astrological chart. Treatment may involve advice about your lifestyle as well as recommendations for medicines made mainly of herbs.

TRAGERWORK ★

This therapy uses gentle manipulation to help you relax. Practitioners claim that the movements used in Tragerwork can also benefit such ailments as high blood pressure, migraines, and asthma.

A Tragerwork practitioner uses his or her hands to find points of tension in your body. The Tragerworker then uses a range of movements—including rocking, gentle stretching, and cradling—to bring about a state of relaxation and a feeling of well-being.

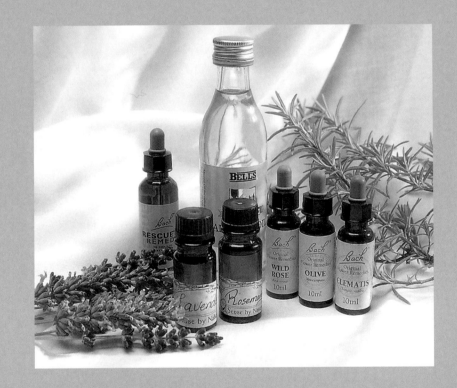